GET **NAKED**

with Your Natural Hair Colour

GET **NAKED**

with Your Natural Hair Colour

Nicole Scott, RHN

Nicole Scott
Registered Holistic Nutritionist
CEO, Own Your Sparkle
www.nicolescott.ca

ISBN 978-1-9990619-0-6 (Paperback)
ISBN 978-1-9990619-1-3 (eBook)
ISBN 978-1-9990619-2-0 (audiobook)

Book production management by Dawn James, Publish and Promote
Edited by Andrea Lemieux
Book Cover design by Franny Armstrong
Cover photograph by Babesclub Boudoir
Perseus Design, Interior Layout & Design

Printed and bound in Canada

I dedicate this book to all the bad-ass Grey-Haired Women who have gone before me. Young or old, you made a choice to go against the norm and say, "This is me." Because you were brave and bold, your actions contributed to a Movement of "Grey Is Okay at Any Age." You inspired me to embrace my sparkle for the health of it and write this book. I am grateful to all my Grey-Haired Heroes, especially my momma bear, Janice.

CONTENTS

CHAPTER ONE

Wake-up Call:
Are You Listening?

"One can choose to go back toward safety or forward toward growth. Growth must be chosen again and again; fear must be overcome again and again."
—ABRAHAM MASLOW

I am lying in the hospital bed and waking up from surgery. I am afraid to look down at my breasts, but I do. They are wrapped in bandages, but I don't see any feminine curves. They have been removed. Chemo and radiation start next week. My heart is heavy knowing it is going to be the biggest battle of my life. Tears are streaming down my face and I look up to see my two teenage girls standing by my side, happy to see me. They hold my hand and Ella says, "It's okay, Mom, you've got this. You're the strongest person I know." My youngest, Sydney, has something on her mind. As I have always encouraged her to speak her truth, even if it's hard, she begins to ask the question that I will never forget: "Mom, you're a nutritionist, you teach prevention.

1

Did you do everything that you knew about to avoid cancer?" I felt a lump in my throat, and as tears poured down my face I looked into her eyes—and then I awoke from my dream! Thank God!

Where did that dream come from? Was it because I had found two lumps in my breasts last year and that had scared the crap out of me? Was it on my mind because I have a friend and teammate going through the same situation? Was it because I was missing a dear family member who left her teenage girls behind—before she turned forty years old— because of cancer? Was it my grandpa or grandma communicating with me from the other side? You see, my grandpa took his own life when I was nineteen years old because the cancer treatment he was going through was unbearable. I was close to my grandpa, and this was the first relative I had lost to cancer who was dear to my heart. His wife, Elsie, my grandma, also died of cancer when I was three years old. She was playful. One memory I have of her is when she was sitting in her wheelchair and I was sitting on her lap. I was playing with a toy gun, firing it off, and she pretended that she was dead. Who was trying to send me a message with this memory? Was Spirit nudging me to ask some deep questions about my own health and how I was treating my body?

Whatever the reason was for that dream, it shook me to my core. That image haunted me. If you are a momma bear, you know the image I am talking about—not being around for your kids for their next birthdays. Then there was the other haunting image of having to truthfully answer Sydney's question and hurting my daughters by telling them, "*No*, I did not do everything I learned in my training. I ignored some of it because I thought it wouldn't happen to me. I do most things right, but I guess I was playing Russian roulette."

Don't we all take chances every day in our lives—driving to work, eating too much processed food, drinking too much alcohol, taking medications, skiing down a hill, going on an adventure? But we don't stop living. We try to live life to the fullest, right? So we listen to that voice in our heads that says stuff such as, "You only live once, so have that shot, drink the vino, eat those chips, purchase that fast food, inject those chemicals in your face, dye that hair, paint those nails," and it goes on and on. We start to justify our poor habits. Why? To fit in with society, to make us feel good, or to convince ourselves in the moment that it's okay. No matter how we justify our decisions, they can add up big time if we aren't careful and impact our health immediately or over time. So that dream, that intuition that I paid attention to, was a wake-up call for me. I have had many wake-up calls on my journey that I will share with you, some I listened to, but with others I wasn't ready for the message and the actions required to deal with them.

What started as a dream, or as some might say, "A message from the Divine," was that nudge for me to start digging deep. It was that nudge that got me writing. Never before have I been forced out of bed with an urge to write. Some mornings it was at four o'clock, and I would write for hours before the house started to wake up. Me? Write? That sounds so hilarious to me. You see, writing has never been a desire of mine. I was never a big reader, and writing, well let's just say I would avoid it if I could. *Coles Notes* in high school and audio books saved me. My handwriting was messy, and my spelling was average. Whoever invented spell-check, I love you! Let's just say it got me through my corporate days. I had spell-check set up before any email went out so I wouldn't embarrass myself. So I am sharing the first of my many insecurities with you in this book. Why? Because I want to show you that we all have them but it's how we deal with them and move past them that count.

The first time my idea to write a book about going grey showed up, I was thirty-five years old. I shelved the idea for years because I had so much *fear*. You know the fear I'm talking about. The fear that paralyzes you from taking action. I dedicate an entire chapter to the topic of fear, which I believe holds us back from living a great life. The point I want to make is that I got a nudge way back to do something, and I allowed fear to win.

Let's shift gears and I'll take you back to my childhood days. I grew up in a small town in Alberta in Western Canada. My grandpa was a cattle rancher, and every Sunday my sister and I would visit him after church to play in the fields, ride horses, look for snakes, and buy a ton of candy from the gas station. Grandpa always used to sneak a quarter into my or my sister's hand without our parents noticing. Twenty-five cents got you a lot of candy back then. I was raised mostly on meat and potatoes with liver on Sundays. My sister and I got caught on many occasions throwing the liver in the toilet or wrapping it in tissue and throwing it in the garbage. Our punishment was no Sunday Disney show. Worst punishment ever, right! Anyone else get caught throwing out their liver? What was your punishment? I don't remember eating a lot of veggies or fruit as a kid; you know, the staples: banana, oranges, apples, canned peas, frozen carrots, and potatoes. Milk was at every meal. I was a thin girl but always seemed to have digestive issues. I was known in the family and my circle of friends as being able to clear a room with a "crop dusting." Not my best trait. There always seemed to be at least one in the family. That was me. I still remember my friends sending me home from school and my mom picking me up because the smell was so bad. I would have saved myself from some very embarrassing moments if I had known what I know now about nutrition.

Did you know that your symptoms are your friends? Are you listening? For years I struggled with digestive and weight issues. I was bulimic all through grade 12. I was the new kid on the block, and I wanted to fit in and be popular. Being thin I thought was the only way to accomplish that. A friend of mine taught me how to do it and helped me keep my weight around 135 pounds while indulging in all the crap I wanted. However, even at that low weight I thought I was fat. My mom caught me, thank goodness, and put the fear in me. That was enough to stop the insanity. My body was screaming at me and I wasn't listening. I would get sick as soon as I slowed down and be out of commission for weeks at a time. I lived at the doctor's, getting the next prescription for antibiotics. The next organ system to start showing symptoms was my respiratory system when I was in my twenties. It appeared that I had environmental allergies. My nose ran all the time, and I always had mucus in my throat to clear. It was annoying but also embarrassing at times. I finally went to the doctor, only to learn that I had postnasal drip and the only way to fix it would be nasal passage surgery. That freaked me out, I was only twenty-seven years old. Surgery, with the risk that it might not work, was not an appealing option. What was I going to do?

The same week I got the news that surgery was my only option, I met an angel. She was a new massage therapist at my chiropractic clinic, and I would book my first of many appointments with her. She started to share stories with me about the connection between dairy allergy and respiratory issues. She had been a nurse for fifteen years before she changed careers. I guess that through her journey working in the hospital she had witnessed the connection. I remember thinking this was a joke. How could milk harm me? I had been raised on it. My parents said it was good for me, and the government said drink your milk daily for stronger bones. Now I have a massage therapist asking me to eliminate all dairy to see if it will help relieve some of my symptoms! This sounded crazy to me, but I had nothing to lose. It seemed like a better option over surgery. My doctor thought it was a crazy idea as well and didn't support my decision. However, against his orders, I would give up my favourite food category for four weeks as an experiment. Guess what? After a few weeks of no dairy, my symptoms started to go away. OMG! My digestive issues started to clear up, my nose stopped dripping 24/7, and no surgery was needed. That was my first *big* wake-up call to the connection between food and symptoms.

Crazy how one food can either harm you or support you. Dairy for me was not a food to help support my body, and I learned that in my twenties. I can't imagine where my health would be if I had not been open to what that amazing woman, my massage therapist, my angel, was telling me.

Like me, my sister had her own issues as a kid. She had a bloated belly and always seemed to have low energy. Her health challenges started to show up aggressively in her twenties with swollen ankles, anemia, and extreme fatigue. For years she would battle with the medical system that was telling her she wasn't eating properly and it was her fault. Even the injections the medical doctors gave her didn't help her. Lucky for her, a friend who was a medical doctor had a cosmetic clinic and wanted to see her as a patient. He was suspicious about her swollen ankles. He started to do his own research and sent her back to her doctor to check for celiac disease. Sure enough, the medical system finally diagnosed her correctly with celiac disease. We were so relieved that we finally knew what was going on in her unhealthy body. It took eight years going through the medical system before she got the right diagnosis.

This experience was a wake-up call for our family. I learned the importance of being *your own health advocate* and to dig deep until you find the root cause of your issue. Be willing to spend money with alternative health professionals such as a naturopathic or a functional medicine doctor to support you on your journey. I strongly believe that everyone needs to invest in a healthcare team so you can hear different opinions, and therefore be able to make an informed decision if you have a health emergency. My sister had suffered for years not being able to live her best life.

I remember going with her over twenty-five years ago to the Canadian Celiac Association in Toronto and learning about her new condition and how we could support her through diet. We learned that to heal her body she would have to stop eating all gluten for the rest of her life. It was an emotional appointment. What would she eat? All of her favourite foods, including beer, bread, and pasta contained gluten. We cried together. As she started to embrace a new way of life, the villi in her digestive tract began to heal. Villi are small finger like projections of tissue found in your small intestine that contain specialized cells that transport nutrients into the bloodstream. When you have celiac disease, the gluten crushes the villi and one can become nutritionally deficient like my sister had. As she started to absorb the nutrients from her gluten-free diet, she began to gain her health back.

There are many resources and tests available now for people to find out quickly if they have celiac disease. No more waiting eight years for a diagnosis like my sister had. If you have celiac disease, lucky for you that the gluten-free options today are 100% better than they were twenty-five years ago. Right, sister? We used to joke that cardboard tasted better than the bread. Thank you for all the amazing bakers who figured out how to make gluten-free bread and pasta taste amazing. My favourite gluten-free bakery is Frankie's, which has an online store that ships all across Canada, and a few retailers carry their products (see the resources section on page 235). You won't be able to tell the difference, I promise.

I want to dive into my first big wake-up call as a new mother. It began with my first born, Ella. Becoming a mother was the biggest "happy story" of my life. Nothing ever prepares you for the *love* you feel for a child. That first time you get to hold your baby and hear their little sounds. You are changed to the core. You want to be better all of sudden. You would do anything and everything to protect your child.

The introduction of my wake-up call was while I was enjoying my maternity leave with my first born. As an infant, Ella would often get sick. Her nose would run constantly, she had itchy ears and shiners under her eyes, and she was often irritable. We had many sleepless nights and we were all exhausted. Ella also had chronic ear infections, which meant many rounds of antibiotics. We were told by the pediatrician that this was normal for a baby. I was lucky enough to get a nudge from a friend to see a naturopathic doctor. A who? I had never heard of this type of doctor before, and I was desperate. That appointment changed our world when we found out that allergies were causing her symptoms. At nine months old, Ella was diagnosed with a ton of food and environmental allergies. I was angry, sad, shocked, and confused. How could this be possible?

I remember feeling sorry for myself, but I was willing to embrace this new life. I would do anything to help her gain better health. As soon as we started removing the allergenic foods from her diet, her body started to heal right in front of our eyes. It was amazing to witness. My learning curve was steep. I had to learn how to live a chemical-free life along with no dairy or gluten. We had a list of seventy-five items that we needed to avoid. Birthday parties were a nightmare for us since Ella seemed to be allergic to everything except fruit and veggies. Why do the worst foods for kids come out at birthday parties? Listen, I'm not judging anyone for their choices because I would probably have served the same junk food at my child's birthday party if it weren't for my wake-up call. You know the junk food I am talking about. Chips, candy from the dollar store, a cake full of sugar and dyes, plus the hot dogs full of fillers on a gluten-laden bun. I have so much compassion for families, and I would like to meet you where you are on your journey. At the time, my husband and I both worked for top processed-food companies. You can probably imagine what our pantry looked like. Before babies, Friday-night dinner was frozen pizza, bagged salad, and store-bought salad dressing. Yikes!

As time went on, I realized Ella's allergies were a gift for me to change my path's direction and move closer to what was to become my mission in life. Who would have thought that Ella would become my reason for change! My second gift showed up seventeen months later—Sydney Jean. I had such a different experience with my second pregnancy because I had educated myself about nutrition and self-care. I gained only twenty-seven pounds vs. the sixty pounds I gained with Ella. I lost all the weight after three weeks of giving birth, had a natural birth (no drugs), and to this day Sydney, age sixteen, has never been on a dose of medication. I was so inspired with our family's positive changes that I decided to leave my corporate career of ten years in the food industry and pursue a new path of holistic nutrition. I registered for a two-year program at the Canadian School of Natural Nutrition five months after Sydney was born. What was I thinking, you ask? Two babies under two and going to night school. Oftentimes I would find myself in the rocker in the middle of the night, boob hanging out, child in arm, and book in lap. As moms, at times we really do try to do it all! A force within us wanting to have more. But I also had a *big why*! I was hungry to help heal Ella so we could have a normal, healthy life. The sacrifice we take on to protect and help our children!

Who stopped dyeing their hair when they were pregnant? Me! Who stopped drinking when they were pregnant? Me! Who started eating better and taking supplements for the first time? Me! Why do we do this? We don't want to harm the baby, and we know these are habits that are potentially dangerous. We don't want to risk it, or do we? Thanks to Dr. Google we can find information about any topic; following are a variety of the opinions I found. What do you think? Do you dye your hair or hold off when you are pregnant?

An article from the Mayo Clinic says that the chemicals in hair dye "aren't generally thought to pose harm to a developing baby. However, given the lack of available evidence, you might consider postponing any chemical hair treatments until after you deliver."[1] And the UK's National Health Service says, "The chemicals in permanent and semi-permanent hair dyes are not highly toxic. Most research, although limited, shows it's safe to colour your hair while pregnant."[2] A story in the *Daily Mail* lists certain hair-dye products that have been banned in the Britain, saying that they "can harm a woman's fertility and endanger her unborn child."[3] However, the American Pregnancy Association says that, "Although fairly limited, most research indicates the chemicals found in both semi-permanent and permanent dyes are not highly toxic and are safe to use during pregnancy. In addition, only small amounts of hair dye may be absorbed by the skin, leaving little that would be able to reach the fetus."[4] And to sum all this up, a group of four doctors reported that there "isn't enough conclusive evidence or research to suggest dying your hair while pregnant will cause harm to your fetus. There have been a few studies linking the use of hair dye to an increased risk of certain types of cancer, but there are also studies that have found no connection at all."[5]

Are you confused? I would be. As I dove deeper into this topic, I found a very important study on chemicals found in the umbilical cords of babies.

In a 2005 study spearheaded by the Environmental Working Group (EWG) in collaboration with Commonweal, researchers at two major laboratories found an average of 200 industrial chemicals and pollutants in umbilical cord blood from 10 babies born in August and September of 2004 in U.S. hospitals. Tests revealed a total of 287 chemicals in the group. The umbilical cord blood of these 10 children, collected by Red Cross after the cord was cut, harbored pesticides, consumer product ingredients, and wastes from burning coal, gasoline, and garbage.

This study represents the first reported cord blood tests for 261 of the targeted chemicals and the first reported detections in cord blood for 209 compounds. Among them are eight perfluorochemicals used as stain and oil repellants in fast food packaging, clothes and textiles—including the Teflon chemical PFOA, recently characterized as a likely human carcinogen by the EPA's Science Advisory Board—dozens of widely used brominated flame retardants and their toxic by-products; and numerous pesticides.

Of the 287 chemicals we detected in umbilical cord blood, we know that 180 cause cancer in humans or animals, 217 are toxic to the brain and nervous system [emphasis mine], and 208 cause birth defects or abnormal development in animal tests. The dangers of pre- or post-natal exposure to this complex mixture of carcinogens, developmental toxins and neurotoxins have never been studied.[6]

Still not sure what to do? What does your gut tell you? Your intuition as a mother? If research shows that babies' umbilical cord blood has 180 cancer-causing toxins in it, it's probably a good idea to cut back where you can. Those numbers are alarming. Is that not a wake-up call as mothers to reduce our chemical load as much as possible? Babies are exposed to major toxins before they are even born. This is not okay. Does that not make you angry? Does it not make you want to investigate why and how? How can I minimize this toxic hit to my unborn baby? These were the types of questions

I had when I found out about Ella's allergies. I wanted answers. My point here is that there is a lot of conflicting information on the internet. It can be confusing when you want to make an informed decision. I didn't have internet at the tip of my fingers eighteen years ago when I was pregnant with Ella. I had to make an informed choice from the information I received from my friends, family, and doctor, and my own intuition. I am glad I listened to my intuition.

I gave up dye and booze for nine months. Over time, those habits started to creep back in. Not sure when and why I thought it was okay to start adding those habits back into my life. Was I not important enough to protect myself from the potential dangers of added toxins? I could go on and on with this one, but I don't want to beat myself up. I was not ready for that kind of change in my life. I told myself that the dye kept me looking youthful and the booze kept me in the game with my social network, or so I thought. Oh, the stories we can make up to justify our choices.

It took me over two years, living in a bubble, to work on healthy living for Ella and for myself. I learned so much and am forever grateful for our journey together to health. She was my teacher. Her story continues in chapter five, where I share more about her healing journey.

Planting the Seed to Grey

May 2018, I took my youngest, Sydney, on a camping trip to Banff National Park with my sister and her hubby, Cameron, and their twin boys. It was that weekend that the seed for me to start moving to the *grey side* began to plant itself. I had long, dark hair, and I wore it up in a bun the entire weekend. My sister commented on the grey hairs that were coming in.

Then the question came, "How often do you dye your hair?" "Every three weeks," I answered. Then Cameron said, "How much do you pay?" I told him around $100 to $150 every three weeks. He started to do the math and said, "Wow that's a lot of money!" I responded sharply, "It's no big deal. I can afford it and I am worth it." Honestly, I got a little defensive. I felt judged, but I let it go. Then what does my sister start doing, she starts looking up funky haircuts on women in their forties with grey hair and showing them to me. "Look at these gorgeous women rocking grey in their forties, Sister. You could totally rock out in *grey*," she says. She started texting me all her favourite pictures. Truth be told, I secretly kept a few of them on my phone. In May 2018 in Banff National Park on a camping trip with my family, the seed was planted. Thank you, Sister! What changed?

Over the months my extra weight around my belly and low energy was starting to draw my attention. I had gained an extra twenty-five pounds—up two pant sizes—and the dreaded muffin top had finally appeared. As a nutritionist, I thought this would never happen to me. I ate well and exercised almost daily. Nothing had changed in my life other than my period. The feelings I had around this weight gain were embarrassment and shame. Thoughts would creep into my mind. What would people think? Why was my body failing me? I was curious about what was happening to my body, which lead me to many discoveries that put me on this new journey.

I knew that, as a nutritionist, I needed to really dig into what was happening to my body and get to root cause. I was listening to the screams my body was sharing. Tender breasts, lumps in my breasts, irregular periods, and rapid weight gain. My symptoms were my friends, and they were telling me something was wrong. My body needed some help. My hope for you, my readers, is that my journey will inspire you to dig deeply into your own health picture and figure out how to achieve the balance your body always craves.

The first thing I did was to reach out to a few of my mentors to ask them for some guidance. Do you have any mentors you trust when it comes to your health? Health experts I mean? Not Dr. Google. Judging by my period tracker during that last year, I was all over the map; things were changing with my hormones big time. I recommend that you track your period as it can provide important information for you and your health professional. I use an app on my phone called "Period Tracker," and so do my girls.

With some great guidance, I knew I needed to start by understanding my hormones. You can test hormones by blood, saliva, and now, urine. I've done blood and saliva before, but never urine. Urine is the newest method that can give you lots of great information to really understand your pathways and dig deeper into the puzzle of hormones. It is more expensive than the other tests, and not covered by healthcare, so be prepared to spend money to get a deeper understanding of your health.

I booked an appointment with my naturopathic doctor, and we agreed that we would start with the DUTCH hormone test. This was a $500 investment for a panel of tests that I paid for out of pocket. I was sent home with the kit and easy instructions to follow. I took five urine samples in a twenty-four-hour period. I dried them out and mailed them off to a lab in California. About two weeks later, I went back to my naturopathic doctor to review the results and discovered that I was estrogen dominant, which I had suspected. Another wake-up call for me! My hormones were out of balance. My levels of estrogen were high, and it showed that I wasn't processing my estrogen properly through the different pathways. The symptoms I was experiencing included rapid weight gain; water retention; irregular periods; tender, lumpy breasts; and low energy. As a nutritionist, I knew elevated estrogen levels are a risk factor for breast and ovarian cancers and may even put you at higher risk of blood clots and stroke. Estrogen dominance may also increase your chances of thyroid dysfunction.

When I had my thyroid markers checked with my medical doctor, they checked for one marker to start with: my TSH. My doctor wouldn't have me tested for the full panel, as I had requested. This was so frustrating as I pay high taxes for this service. If your TSH looks normal, no more testing happens, which is what happened to me. I learned that you can have a normal TSH reading but your other five markers could still be out of balance. If you, my reader, have gone to your doctor and had only one marker tested, demand a full thyroid panel to see the entire picture. If your doctor won't issue you a full panel, then your naturopathic doctor can get you one. A great book to understand your thyroid better is *The Paleo Thyroid Solution* by Elle Russ (see the resources section on page 235). This book was a huge awakening for me and it empowered me more than ever to stay on top of my thyroid health. I started listening to podcasts and reading more books on this topic. I was back in school and more motivated than ever to learn how to gain optimal health. Two colleagues whom I admire in the field of holistic health are Jenn Pike and Samantha Gladish (See the resources section). They specialize in women's hormones and have great podcasts and online programs to empower you to take control of your health.

My naturopathic doctor (ND) put me on a program to reduce my estrogen levels. It started with weekly IV drips to help detoxify and push out the estrogen. During my first drip, I couldn't keep my eyes open and I fell asleep right away. Sitting in a comfy reclined leather chair with the warm sun on my face, I was out. I felt the way a cat must feel on a sunny day by a window. I woke up an hour and half later, and for the next twenty-four hours all I did was go to the bathroom. The treatment was really flushing me out in a good way and I knew it was helping. I would go back a number of times over the months for continued support. I was so fascinated by the way the body works and the fact that there were tools available that could support me beyond my healthful diet.

I was also prescribed supplements of iron, glutathione, and vitamin B12 for estrogen support, and I continued taking a whole-food plant concentrate in capsule form called Juice Plus+. I began taking these amazing plant concentrates fourteen years ago, and they were a key element to Ella's healing and to a new career path for me in network marketing—about which I will share later.

In the meantime, I also had live blood analysis done by another naturopath, and I continue to have this done to this day. I love this form of analysis as you get to immediately see the state of your health. It is amazing what our blood can tell us about our health. European doctors use this tool as part of their protocol to treat patients, and I am a big fan of it. Imagine if our medical doctors could start to use this tool to help support better health. My vision of the future would be to have my tax dollars put towards a medical system that supports prevention and healthcare not just "sick care."

During this appointment, I asked my ND to check my breasts as they were feeling lumpy, and there were a few new bumps that I was concerned about. She checked them over and was concerned and said I should have my medical doctor do the same. Well, I left that appointment with some fear brewing in me: What if? There was no breast cancer in my family, so I was sure it was nothing to worry about; it was just extra precaution. I went the same day to the walk-in clinic. There was a female doctor on call and she checked me over. She was suspicious as well, and wanted me to get checked out ASAP. This was the first time, at age forty-seven, when I had ever had to have my breasts checked out for something. I have been doing monthly self-checkups for years, but this time seemed different. There were unfamiliar bumps that even I was suspicious about.

I decided I would not get a mammogram, but instead I would begin with an ultrasound exam. If it looked abnormal, I would go back to get the mammogram. I had to wait over the weekend and into the middle of the next week before I got the results. OMG! Have you ever had to wait that long for a test result? You can drive yourself *crazy* telling yourself stories that can put you into a never-ending "what if" state. I ended up calling the doctor and getting the results over the phone. I took a deep breath, and then I was told they were just cysts and no need to worry. Phew! That was a very scary phone call. We never want to hear the cancer word. That experience got me diving into my own health even deeper. Another wake-up call for me!

What else could I be doing to support my body? What causes estrogen dominance? What else could I be doing to reduce estrogen in my body? Back to the books I went.

The great thing about being a part of a "health community" is you get to hear about a variety of holistic ideas and solutions. I love being part of many online Facebook groups that keep me connected and informed about holistic living. I started to see a few posts about DNA tests, and even DNA-customized supplements. Say what? This idea was so cool to me. I dove in to learn more. I found an old colleague who was connected to a Toronto-based company that was on the cutting edge of DNA research and customizing supplements to support your body. After some research and a great discussion with her, this became my next move to optimizing my health. How much would you be willing to invest to feel your best? I was willing to do what it took to get to the root cause of my symptoms. I wanted to feel awesome again.

My DNA kit arrived. I provided a saliva sample and sent it back to the company, and they mailed it to McGill University for full analysis. I waited anxiously for about two months to get the results. When my package arrived in the mail, I was excited but also nervous about what my DNA would tell me. There was no turning back. I was going to have to own my DNA story. I was going to empower myself with this information. I opened up my forty-five-page report and studied it for a few hours, placing sticky notes all over it and writing down a ton of questions. I jumped on the phone the same week to talk with a top ND at the company, Dr. Bryce Wylde. He was amazing explaining what it all meant. My report card was an eight out of ten, so not bad. Thanks, Mom and Dad. However, there were a few areas to take a look at and begin to support daily. My DNA story confirmed that the weaknesses in my body included detoxification pathways, estrogen pathways, poor dairy metabolism, and a slow metabolizer of stimulants such as coffee. I felt empowered with this information because it could help me put more of the puzzle pieces together. I knew from a young age that coffee and I did not fit. I would always get the red cheeks and coffee jitters, so I had stayed away from coffee and it never became a habit. I had the same experience with alcohol, and I wish I had been as motivated to stay away from it as a teen, but that had not been the case. I had discovered dairy as a culprit to my gut issues in my twenties, so I stayed away from it most of the time. As I was going through my journey and listening to the clues, I had already discovered what my DNA test was telling me; I just didn't have an official report. The body always gives us symptoms as clues to whether or not it is happy. The question is, *are we quiet enough to listen?*

The first two weeks on the customized supplements was flushing me out big time. I have never peed so much in my life. I lost about ten pounds those first few weeks, so I knew this formula was working for me. The formula was helping me flush out daily toxins and giving more support to the pathways that were jammed. My tender breasts went away, and the lumps in my breasts were coming down. Wow! These customized supplements were making a difference in my health. I felt as though I had my breasts back. Ladies, if you have ever had such tender breasts that no one can touch them, you know what I am talking about. I'm so grateful I paid attention and discovered this amazing tool to better support my health.

Last summer, before my customized supplements arrived, I spent a lot of time researching other things I could be doing to bring down my estrogen symptoms. I thought I was doing a good job living a healthy lifestyle, but obviously I still had areas to improve. We all have room for improvement, would you not agree? Where in your life could you be working on reducing the toxic load to improve your health? I had three big habits to address: alcohol, hair dye, and nail polish and gel nails. Why was I so resistant to changing them? I had strong stories attached to each of them that I slowly had to change and focus on my bigger "why"! Let's talk about the last three habits I finally parted ways with.

1. Alcohol

Let's talk about alcohol, or as I like to call it, "the drink." I love a great glass of wine or two or three when out with friends. This was a habit that had a strong hold on me. I knew this habit was not serving my body well, yet I was still doing it. As I researched more about the impact alcohol was having in my body, I started to pay attention. Here are some insights I discovered that really got me thinking differently:

A review of the scientific evidence linking alcohol consumption, estrogen, and breast cancer risk showed that alcohol can change the way a woman's body metabolizes estrogen (that is, how estrogen works in the body). The studies found that alcohol can cause blood estrogen levels to rise, which can lead to increased cell proliferation and a greater opportunity for genetic damage.[7]

An article in *ScienceDaily* reported on a study published in the journal *PLOS ONE* that stated: "When estrogen levels are higher, alcohol is much more rewarding. ... Women may be more vulnerable to the effects of alcohol or more likely to overindulge during certain stages of their cycle when estrogen levels are higher, or may be more likely to seek out alcohol during those stages."[8]

The American Cancer Society States: "Most people know that heavy drinking can cause health problems. But many people might not know that drinking alcohol also can raise their risk of getting cancer,"[9] and cancers that have been linked to alcohol use include mouth, throat, voice box, esophagus, liver, colon and rectum, and breast. "For each of these cancers, the more alcohol you drink, the higher your cancer risk."[10]

I already had high estrogen. I thought that consuming alcohol could have been a contributing factor to my rising estrogen levels, health problems, and extra weight gain. I was listening! Next I discovered that when the number of drinks you consume per day goes up, so does your risk of cancer. A meta-analysis of 53 studies, where the data from multiple studies is analyzed, found that for each alcoholic drink consumed per day, the relative risk of breast cancer increased by about 7%. Women who had 2 or 3 alcoholic drinks per day had a 20% higher risk of breast cancer compared to women who didn't drink alcohol.[11]

When you factor in my drinking habit, my DNA results, and some of my lifestyle choices, I knew I needed to make changes for my future self. Remember I told you I lost two grandparents to cancer, so I was really starting to pay attention to this information.

A big wake-up call for me was the overwhelming research on how alcohol levels impacted estrogen and the risk of cancer. Holy crap! I am sure I read about it in my nutritional studies. I even coach women to reduce their alcohol consumption for better health. Yet I have played the dance with alcohol since I was fourteen years old. I drank way too much as a teen and that carried into my adult life. It became almost a daily habit. Where do habits come from? Where do we get sold on the idea that drinking is fun and cool? We are bombarded by TV ads and magazines and pressured at times by our social crowd that drinking is where it's at. We get sold on believing that if you don't drink you are missing out. We see others do it daily, and then we think it's okay and we do it too. My dad was a daily beer drinker. After my parents' divorce, my mom became a big drinker and loved to party. It was part of my lifestyle growing up. As a kid growing up, when you see that behaviour daily you think it's normal. For some of us as adults, it eventually becomes *our* normal. I abused it many times in my life, especially when my marriage was breaking down. I would sneak in a bottle of wine before my husband would come home so I could function better—or so I thought. That was just a lie I told myself. A year after the divorce and the daily drink was getting old, I knew I needed to do something different. I was coaching hundreds of people monthly on a whole-foods challenge that involved many lifestyle principles; one of them was no drinking for thirty days. That scared the crap out of me. I don't think I have ever abstained from drinking for thirty days since I was a teen, other than when I was pregnant. That is scary when you think about it. I was programmed and had created a habit so big that it was part of me.

Finally, in September 2016, after kids got off to school for a new term, I made a commitment to stop drinking for thirty days. I needed to be that role model for my clients, for my family, for my friends, for my kids, and most importantly, for myself. I was doing everything else right: no dairy, no wheat, stop eating past 6 p.m., move daily, drink lots of water, add whole-plant concentrates, have two shakes a day, and do not consume processed foods. I did all of that perfect-ly, but now I was ready to say no to the *drink*. I learned to drink fizzy water and make spritzers. I also enjoyed a varie-ty of herbal teas. Guess what happened? I accomplished my goal. No drink for thirty days and the bonus was I dropped fourteen pounds and felt amazing. Wow! Who would have thought that alcohol was making me fat, but it was! Now that I understand my DNA weakness this makes sense to me. I suck at processing alcohol in my system. Yes, I would be the one with a three-day hangover if I drank too much. I could never understand how I had friends who could do it over and over and over again with no symptoms. I could never keep up with my friends. One big night and I was screwed for days. But I loved to party, stay up late, and keep up with the crowd, only to pay the price for days afterwards. Oh, the dreaded hangovers—I do not miss them! I realized that I was doing so much harm to my body yet trying to fit into the crowd. What price was I paying for the drink?

Where are you on the path of the drink? Do you drink daily? Socially? Where did that habit come in? Why do you drink? Were your parents big drinkers? What is it about the drink you enjoy? Is it impacting your wellbeing? How many times in a year do you wake up hungover? Do you think you process it well? These are important questions to ask. Again, remember, my motivation was the fact that I had lumps in my breasts at age forty-seven. My life flashed before me. What if? It is amazing what motivates you to start changing your *stinking thinking* and your habits that do not serve you well. My drinking habit has changed drastically. I can go months without a drink now and can say *no* to the drink at parties. I rarely have alcohol in my house unless I am having guests over to entertain. If you are a drinker, I dare you to abstain from drinking for thirty days and see how it makes you feel. Not going to lie, the first few weeks test you, big time! In the beginning I stayed away from social drinking settings to avoid the temptation, but once you get past those hard days, they do get easier. A book I read called *This Naked Mind* by Annie Grace (see the resources section on page 235) really helped me understand what the drink was doing to my body and my brain. I joined the author's private Facebook group for some motivation as well. You can do anything for thirty days; I dare you. If I can do it, so can you!

2. Hair Dye

Another habit that was not contributing to my best health was dyeing my hair every three weeks. When I started to deep dive on what the big deal was, I came across more information that would inspire me to go to the *grey* side. I will share more of those details in chapter three when we dive into "What's Hiding in Your Hair Dye?"

After researching, I knew in my heart that not only did I need to cut back significantly on my drinking, but I also had to stop dyeing my hair. Since I knew my DNA weaknesses, I knew I needed to make the next move. October 12, 2018, was my last application of root touch-up. I decided to work towards blending my greys, which meant I had to start highlighting over many appointments. I had researched several different ways to go grey, and blending seemed to be the best option for me. I will share more of my journey on this process later.

3. Nail Polish and Gel Nails

Next on my list to detox my life was nail polish! Yep, full of chemicals to impact estrogen—another toxin I was willing to depart with after learning what it was doing to my hormones. "The so-called toxic trio of nail polish consists of dibutyl phthalate (a plasticizer), toluene (to evenly suspend color), and formaldehyde (a known carcinogen that is used as a hardening agent). ... According to the EPA, this chemical appears to have relatively low acute (short-term) and chronic (long-term) toxicity."[12] "Researchers have linked hormone disruptors such as TPHP to early onset of puberty, neurodevelopmental problems and obesity."[13] To think I was doing this every few weeks in the name of vanity. Yikes!

I used to get my nails and toes done every two weeks. These toxins can leach into your body. You see, I was a nail-biter my entire life, and I was always embarrassed by how horrible my nails looked. After my divorce, I was determined to treat myself to nice nails. I had gels on my nails for over three years and polish on my toes. When I realized that this was another level of toxicity that was entering my body, I knew they had to go. No more polish. I have been free of polish for four months and know it is for the better. I do miss it, and how fancy it made me look, but again, I am so clear on my *why*. My short natural nails are starting to grow on me. The best part, I don't bite them anymore.

This is what I learned about gel nails: A dermatologist, Dr. Adigun, certified by the American Academy of Dermatology, says that "UV exposure during gel manicures should be a concern for everyone, not just people who know they are especially UV-sensitive, because the lamps used in these manicures emit UVA rays. Although these rays don't burn the skin like UVB rays, ... they do penetrate the skin to damage DNA and collagen, which can lead to premature aging and may increase skin cancer risk."[14]

I am glad I said goodbye to the polish. It has taken a full four months to have my real nails grow out and look healthy again, but it was worth the wait. Will I put polish on my nails ever again? I don't know, maybe for a special occasion, but for now I am polish free.

Other Hazards Lurking in the Home

Monthly root touch-ups gone. Check! Alcohol reduced significantly. Check! No more nail treatments. Check! Now the next step was to check the chemical load in my house. Where else was it showing up? My makeup was about 75% organic, but I knew I could still improve on that. I threw out everything nonorganic and replaced it with clean-ingredient makeup. I have a great health-food store called Natural Solutions in town that I have been supporting for eleven years. I am grateful for their service to our community. Yes, clean and organic products cost more money, but again, I was willing to invest. As Dr. Sears says, "Pay now or pay later." I have also noticed that I tend to wear less makeup and go more natural these days, which also feels very freeing.

Do you worry about the chemicals on your produce? You should because they are heavily sprayed with pesticides and herbicides, some more than others. I printed out the list of the Environmental Working Group's 2018 "Shopper's Guide to Pesticides in Produce" to cut down on the level of chemicals that were still sneaking into our fridge and into our bodies. You can find a current guide by going to their website (see the resources section on page 235). The number of organic fruits and vegetables in my small rural town is limited. I buy a lot of organic frozen produce through the winter instead of the overripe, well-travelled produce that is heavily sprayed.

I also learned that industrial pollutants of nearly all kinds almost always have estrogen-mimicking properties, which add to the estrogen load. Do you use plastic products in your household? We still had plastics in our house, and I was still drinking out of plastic water bottles. Now I know better. Chemicals in plastics have been proven to disrupt our hormones and increase estrogen in our bodies. "Polyvinyl chloride, or PVC, is widely known as the most toxic plastic for health and the environment. In its production, it releases dioxins, phthalates, vinyl chloride, ethylene dichloride, lead, cadmium and other toxic chemicals."[15] See the resources section on page 235 for "Made Safe," a great website to learn how to cut down on plastics and other toxins in household and personal-care products.

One study of interest found that the "[m]akers of water bottles ... now sell products that don't contain BPA, a chemical that can mimic the sex hormone estrogen. But a new study says that even if they don't contain BPA, most plastic products release estrogenic chemicals."[16]

Another change my family needed to make was to substitute plastic for glass. We now have more glass containers for storing food in the fridge, and we have replaced most plastic water bottles with stainless steel or glass. I even have a ceramic tea mug that I use when I travel, and I love it.

My family isn't perfect, but we are aware of what to eliminate to be healthier. We work on keeping the toxic load low. It is easy for toxins to sneak their way in. Let's face it, we live in a toxic world. Our air is polluted, our drinking water is chemically treated (chlorine and fluoride), and our food is sprayed with chemical cocktails. Last week my new couch arrived and I had it sprayed with tons of chemicals just in case the cats pee on it, but I paid the price of a house full of toxins. Ugh! The man spraying it had to wear a mask, and I opened all the windows and made everyone leave the house for hours. A trade-off at times. Do my teens love and eat junk food? Heck yes! It shows up more than I would like but they know better. I guess they need to have their own stories and wake-up calls—hopefully not as many as I did. As you can see, I have made some huge changes to my personal habits and my family's. I feel as though I have reduced my chemical load significantly, and the result is that I feel much healthier. My energy has bounced back, napping is no longer mandatory, and my breast tenderness is gone. My weight is slowly coming off as well. These are all signs that my body is getting healthier, which was my goal.

There you have it, dear readers: my *why* to writing this book. I want to attain optimal health for me, and I want optimal health for you too. What are the places where you can commit to reducing your toxic load? Are you after optimal health like I am? How far will you go? We are all on a journey. Along the journey we can have a few wake-up calls or many. It's up to us to choose to listen to them or not. I am glad I had enough wake-up calls and started to pay attention to the whispers. It inspired me to be vulnerable and share from my heart my journey to gaining better health.

I invite you to come along on our "Gorgeous-Grey Movement" and see if you can get to a place where you can *own that sparkle* and create your *new health story* like I did. The movement has started and I am so glad I get to share it with you.

CHAPTER TWO

How the Media Impacts Your Hair-Colour Choices

"Don't you dare compare your magic to mine or anyone else's. That's a fool's mission, you know. No happiness was ever born wishing you had someone else's gifts while ignoring your own. Stop looking around and look within. You are magic, wild woman. Own that thing."

—Brooke Hampton

Did you know that by 2015, 75% of American women colour their hair compared with only 7% in 1950?[1] Shocker! This fact fascinates me. A new billion-dollar category emerged, and we women bought into it. I was curious. What and who contributed to this explosive growth over close to seventy years? In my opinion, many factors impacted this growth, including increasing acceptance, safer product offerings, social media influence, Hollywood, peer pressure, and changing lifestyles. Before I dive in and discuss each of these areas, let's first take a peek into the history of hair dye and find out how it became mainstream.

History

From ancient Egypt to modern-day America, hair colour has been a consistent beauty trend. Our methods and options have changed dramatically throughout history, but the interest in the potential of hair colour remains unchanged. Ancient Egyptians were among the first known people to use hair dye, applying henna to darken greying hair and to paint their fingernails. What is henna? Henna is made from the dried leaves of the tropical henna plant, and it has been used for thousands of years as a dye to colour the hair and to decorate the body. For ancient Egyptians, appearance was important and remains so today in our modern-day world. Appearance indicated a person's status, role in a society, or political significance. Egyptian and modern-day hairstyles have a lot in common. Like modern hairstyles, Egyptian hairstyles varied with age, gender, and social status. Later, during ancient Greek and Roman times, people used different methods and ingredients for dyeing their hair, including berries, crushed nutshells, and vinegar as well as henna. The first permanent hair colour was jet black and made from leeches mixed with vinegar. Other civilizations used hair colour to show their rank and frighten the enemy on the battlefield. During the Roman Empire, prostitutes were required to have yellow hair to indicate their profession, but most of them wore wigs. In several cultures, prostitutes were forced to wear different colours from most of the populace to distinguish themselves from the "respectable" women. Not much changed until the 1800s when the British chemist William Henry Perkin made an accidental discovery that changed hair dye forever. "In an attempt to generate a cure for malaria … [Perkins] created the first synthesized dye out of coal tar in the year 1863. The color was mauve, so [it was] named Mauveine. Soon after, his chemistry professor August Hoffman derived a color-changing molecule from Mauveine (called para-phenylenediamine, or PPD), and it remains the foundation for most permanent hair dyes today."[2]

In 1907, French chemist Eugene Schueller took PPD and created the first hair colour for commercial purposes, and it became known as L'Oréal. L'Oréal has become the world's largest cosmetics company today and has expanded business in the beauty segment in hair colour, skin care, sun protection, makeup, perfume, haircare, and men's skincare. Many top hair companies followed suit, including Garnier, Aveda, Redken, and Clairol, capturing market share as they developed competing hair products. Hair colours are considered cosmetic products that are used primarily to change the colour of hair. The main reason people have dyed their hair was to cover the grey; however, currently it is often used as a fashion statement. Hair colouring can be done at home or professionally at a spa or hair salon. With more women in the workforce and having limited free time, many are opting for the convenient home kit for root touch ups and full colour, which they can do in less than an hour—with no babysitter required. New hair colour technology provides easier, gentler, faster, and more convenient options, making it more attractive to the consumer and helping drive sales. Who would have thought that the advances in hair colour in the 1900s, would turn into a beauty phenomenon that continues today?

Hollywood[3,4,5]

Do you think Hollywood plays an important part influencing women's hair colour and style choices? Heck *yes! Scroll through history by the decade and you will see the big stars who had a huge impact on the way women coloured and styled their hair.*

1920s
Jet black was the preferred hair shade thanks in part to actress Louise Brooks. Women had to sneak into hair salons because dyed hair was deemed taboo.

1930s
You can thank Howard Hughes (and Jean Harlow) for the platinum blonde beauty trend. In 1931, Hughes released a film called *Platinum Blonde*, where Jean Harlow dyed her hair an icy-coloured hue. Harlow would dye her hair once a week, saying that if it weren't for her hair, Hollywood wouldn't know she was alive. Many fans quickly followed suit, dyeing their hair to match Harlow's. American women used peroxide and laundry bleach to emulate ultra-blonde. Jean Harlow died at age twenty-seven due to kidney failure. Some speculate that her weekly dye job contributed to her death.

1940s
Darker hair comes back into style because of rationing during WWII. Katherine Hepburn and Ava Gardner were two major fashion and beauty icons at the time.

1950s
Marilyn Monroe makes platinum blonde trendy again. Before 1950, going blonde involved bleach and a lot of damage.

Then everything changed for the hair industry. Clairol would introduce a revolutionary one-step hair dye product that could be used at home and that actually lightened hair without bleaching it. This new easy-to-use product became a hit with the masses as women still preferred not to publicize the fact that they coloured their hair. "Hair color so natural only her hairdresser knows for sure" was Clairol's advertisement campaign at the time.

1960s

Highlights became the trend when Audrey Hepburn wore them in the famous movie *Breakfast at Tiffany's*. Clairol launched the first Frost & Tip in-home highlighting kit. By the late 1960s, colouring one's hair was mainstream, and 1968 was the last year Americans were asked to state their hair colour on passports—the prevalence of hair dye made this information pointless.

1970s

Frosting became popular, giving a natural sun-kissed look. One-third of American women were dying their hair now, and public acceptance was growing. Slogans such as L'Oréal's "Because you're worth it" encouraged acceptance of openly using hair-colour products.

1980s

This decade was all about experimenting with hair. Rock star Madonna made growing-out roots cool, and the punk rock scene brought crazy colours to store shelves. Celebrity endorsements began and companies started securing some of the biggest names in Hollywood, such as Cybill Shepherd and Heather Locklear. This was a natural progression as Hollywood stars had been inspiring hair colour trends since the 1930s.

1990s

Chunky highlighted stripes became trendy and punk and rock influences continued, which is where the 100% vegan, cruelty free brand Unicorn Hair first originated.

2000s

The ombré hair-colouring effect becomes the most popular trend in Hollywood. This is where hair gradually gets lighter towards the ends.

2010s

Thanks to social media and risk-taking celebrities, new colour trends emerge such as rainbow, grey and rose. As you scroll through social media looking for inspiration, you will find several support groups and websites that help women transition to grey. It is a beautiful movement that is happening, and brave women are showing their natural beauty, and inspiring others in the process. To the women who have gone before me, I say thank you. Not only did you give me the courage to ditch the dye, but also to start my own online movement called the "Gorgeous Grey Movement."

A big shoutout to Hollywood celebrities Rachel McAdams, Glenn Close, Jessica Biel, Helen Mirren, Katie Holmes, and Jamie Lee Curtis, to name a few, who have been spotted on the red carpet embracing a trend that was once—their grey hair! It was rare to see stars without a head of perfectly coloured hair, but times are changing thanks to these bold, confident women. We are starting to see stars proudly showing their completely grey hair, or showing their roots. This is huge, folks! This is sending such a powerful message to all women that *grey is okay! You are okay. Growing old is okay, and we don't need to hide it. We are still worthy and adding value to society. Our grey does not define us—or does it?*

Double Standard[6]

Why is there such a double standard for going grey? Men seem to embrace grey with a lot more ease than women. Why is that? Where does this double standard come from? We need to take a good look at the different roles that men and women have played for thousands of years.

Reflecting back in history, remember that the primary function for women was to attract a mate and reproduce. The average life expectancy one hundred years ago was about forty-eight years, so women died before they had much grey hair. Hence, there was a strong association between loss of fertility and a woman's value to society and the appearance of grey hair. For centuries this message has been hard-wired into the brains of men and women. The good news is that these old programmed stories have been changing since the feminist revolution. Our role as women has expanded more than ever, and we are living longer (worldwide average: 72 years, Canada: 83.9 years, USA: 81.1 years[7]); US statistics show that American women work outside the home more (32.7% in 1948 vs. 56.8% 2016[8]); in Canada, women have babies later in life (average age 26.7 in the mid-1970s[9] vs. 30.8 in 2016[10]), and we are more educated than ever.

In the early 1970s, when dyes and chemicals became popular, hair colouring became a routine for women to avoid feeling old and less valued. The TV commercials had us believing we needed to dye our hair to be sexy and wanted by a man. Take a few minutes and Google hair commercials from the 1970s and, like me, you will probably want to throw up. We sure have come a long way, women. Well done!

Now let's talk about the primary function of men in our society. They have been the protectors and breadwinners. They would hunt for food and protect their tribe. A man's value for thousands of years was based on having power and strength. Having some salt-and-pepper or white hair didn't impact their role in society. A century ago, men with white hair was a sign of distinction, hinted at nobility, and was even a sign of masculinity. Today men's roles have not changed much, nor has the way society views their white hair. They are still expected to bring home the bacon, protect their families, and guide their children towards success. Grey hair for men has always been accepted by society, and that still seems to be the case today.

I find men with salt-and-pepper or grey hair to be sexy. It screams confidence and boldness. Role models for men have shown up in Hollywood, including Richard Gere, Sean Connery, and Brad Pitt. Remember back in 2006 when *People magazine featured George Clooney as the sexiest man alive with his salt-and-pepper look. But I bet you couldn't find one magazine back then featuring a woman who displayed the same look, and that was only thirteen years ago. With new technology and new paradigm shifts, change is inevitable, which means we have to adapt to new ways of thinking, new ways of seeing each other, and new ways of accepting the new and different. As more women say yes to their natural sparkle, their brave act will influence many. It will send a powerful message to the world. "This is me!" "I don't need to hide!" "Our health is worth it!" "We are worth it!" I can't wait to see more healthy, sexy, grey-haired women walking the grocery stores, making covers of magazines, and walking the red carpet.*

Peer Pressure

Would you not agree that most of us want to fit in with the crowd? Heck *yes!* Why is that? Because it feels good and safe. As human beings we have basic needs to fulfill for survival. Maslow's hierarchy of needs explains that our basic needs must be met first before we can reach the highest level, called self-actualization. One of the basic needs is love and belongingness. The need for acceptance (belonging) is a basic human instinct, and some value it more than others. We all want to fit in. To achieve that, we often wear different masks, depending on the environment and whom we are with. We might have numerous versions of ourselves—for home, or at work, or even on our social media platforms. All edited and tweaked to be accepted in that particular situation. The question is, are we being accepted for who we truly are, or merely for the version we choose to present of ourselves? What mask do you choose to wear for the world? What if you could wear the "mask" that represented your true self? How would you feel? Would it be freeing? Would it be risky? What would it look like? I have worn many masks over the years to "fit in" and feel loved. How about you?

When do we start to put the different masks on to fit in? Think back to high school or even grade school. You will remember the few kids who stood out in class. They dressed differently, they wore their hair differently, and they just had an "I don't care what you think, here I am" attitude. I secretly admired these kids from afar, imagining how cool it would be not to worry about others' opinions. As a kid I remember judging the "weird kids," just as everyone else did. Their weirdness was what everyone talked about, and that scared me. I didn't want to be the kid everyone talked about in a negative way because that would be so embarrassing and uncomfortable. I just wanted to fit in and be part of the cool crowd. To feel loved. Can anyone relate to this? The desperation of fitting in makes you do stupid stuff, such as stealing brand-name clothes because you can't afford them. I got caught stealing clothes and was charged in grade 9. That was the scariest moment I recall in high school, having to deal with a cop and my mom at the same time. OMG! What stupid things have you done to fit in with the crowd? If I could go back in time and give advice to my younger self I would say, "Just be you and don't worry about fitting in all the time. Different is good. It makes you stand out from the crowd, and in today's world we need more people to stand out and make a difference." Going grey stands out today, especially when you do it before age fifty. It says to the world, "I am okay with my natural beauty. I will not be defined by magazines, YouTube channels, and Hollywood trends. I own my sparkle." A big shoutout to my sparkle friends who decided to say yes and go against society's expectations. You are part of a new movement where we are defining our own beauty. Think of the ripple effect we will have on future generations.

Industry:

The global haircare industry is expected to reach US$211.1 billion by 2025.[11] Specifically, the hair-colour segment is expected to grow year over year by over 8%,[12] driven by millenniums choosing novelty colours such as blue, orange, yellow, and purple. Who drives this trend? Consumers use hair colour and dye not only to cover grey hair but also to make a fashion statement. Consumers' desire to look fashionable, along with celebrity endorsements, drive hair-colour sales. The testimonial of a popular celebrity adds instant credibility to a company's hair product. Monkey see monkey do. Advertisements on television, social-media platforms, and other media have a large impact on the potential consumers.

The segment of chemical hair products dominates the global market because of the availability of a large range of colours that are offered at a low cost. Look at any flyer today, and you will see that you can pick up a hair dye for under five dollars. However, excessive use of chemicals in hair colours is expected to hamper growth of the target market in the near future as more women are choosing natural beauty products. Development of different types of natural, organic, and non-chemical colours and botanicals can create new opportunities for players in the global market. I will discuss more on natural products and the trends in chapter four.

This trend reminds me of a time over ten years ago when I witnessed the food industry starting to wake up to consumers' demands for healthier products. They wanted fewer toxic and more organic products at a reasonable price. We slowly began to see a shift in companies developing healthier options and more consumers were buying organic products. The Organic Trade Association reported that 81% of families with children sometimes purchase organic products.

Their reported reasons included better health and the desire to avoid toxic pesticides and fertilizers. Some parents said they wanted to reduce their family's exposure to genetically modified organisms (GMOs) and growth hormones.[13] This was a huge shift in the food industry, and companies have had to adapt because consumers demanded it. I believe we are now witnessing the same shift in the beauty industry as well. Consumers are demanding healthier options because they realize that what they put on their bodies is just as important as the food they eat. Some excellent books have been published that expose the beauty industry and have brought a new awareness of the toxins hiding in our bathrooms. For example, *Not Just a Pretty Face: The Ugly Side of the Beauty Industry, There's Lead in Your Lipstick: Toxins in Our Everyday Body Care and How to Avoid Them*, and *Toxic Beauty*. (Please see the resources section on page 235.)

The beauty industry is shifting slowly, and I believe in the next ten-plus years it will look very different. I predict that we will see more women embracing grey at a younger age, and more consumers demanding healthier options. Why? Because cancer statistics showed that in 2017, 1 in 2 Canadians would be diagnosed with cancer.[14] People are scared. People are waking up. People want better health. People are demanding different alternatives. People are expecting better from companies. Something has to change for us to have healthier bodies, so let's start by reducing the toxic load!

BareMinerals founder and beauty "Nostradamus" Leslie Blodgett spoke at a convention in 2015 about the future of the industry, and when asked what she thought was the most interesting beauty trend, she said that there was a split in how women approached beauty: Many women have procedures done in doctors' offices, and yet there is a trend toward being more self-compassionate and accepting of themselves as they are. When asked how she thought women would react to changes in the industry, she said that she believes women will continue to feel that the new technologies are safe and effective. Regarding hair dye, she pointed out that at first it wasn't accepted, but now it is almost expected. She stated that women want to stay healthy and active, saying, "I think the health and well-being movement is here to stay.[15]

This is exciting news to hear about beauty trends. I love that she states, "I think the health and well-being movement is here to stay." This gives me hope that the work I have been doing for the past fourteen years as a holistic nutritionist is setting people up for a healthier future, which fills my soul purpose.

Social-Media Beauty Trends Today

Did you know that in 2019 L'Oréal and Vogue declared Grey Hair the Hottest Shade of the Year? Grey has become so popular that social-media site Pinterest even says that searches for the phrase "color grey" has increased by 879% in the last year alone.[16] According to a press release, Orrea Light, Vice President of L'Oréal global marketing product development and beauty innovation, says that "it's the hottest shade of the year. Although it's taken years for people to realize just how great the color grey is, it looks like the shade is here to stay. Not only has silver hair been a top color trend on the runways and it is the 'it' color for women of all ages, we love what the color stands for—it symbolizes charisma, ethereal energy, power, focus and it is beyond chic."[17]

Several hair companies have jumped on board and launched in-home products to cater to this grey trend. For example, L'Oréal has launched three in-home silver shades that include Smokey Silver, Soft Silver, and Silver Blue. Is grey the new blonde, and is it here to stay? You can't go on social media today without been exposed to a woman who is embracing grey or dying their hair grey. Furthermore, "*Glamour* U.K. reported that according to a survey of 2017 hair trends by L'Oréal Professional, 28 percent of the women included in its research are embracing or considering silver hair."[18]

Jump on Instagram and search #greyhair, and you will find 1,832,854 tags; #grannyhair, 341,748 tags; #greyhair-dontcare, 238,966 tags; and #grombre, 39,750 tags. Accounts on Instagram that focus on grey hair have a huge following, such as Grombre at 115,000 followers. Then jump over to Facebook, where you can do a search and find several grey support groups to help you with your transition. Some groups are as large as 25,000 members supporting each other on the path to natural grey. There is no doubt that beauty consumers are increasingly turning to their peers for advice on trends influenced by online social-media platforms such as YouTube, Instagram, Twitter, Pinterest, and Facebook. I would like to think that this is more a *movement* than a trend. I believe "natural grey" is here to stay as more women embrace being their authentic selves.

Today, hair dye products make up a large percentage of the beauty industry's revenue. Clairol research reports that the 71% of women who dye their hair do so to "look and feel more attractive."[19] According to Marcy Cona, Clairol's in-house creative director of colour and style, women want to "live the fantasy that they're still 30 or 35 instead of 45 or 60."[20] Then we have celebs like Katy Perry and Emma Stone, who love to surprise us with their drastic colour changes, and the pastel movement going strong, it seems like experimenting with hair colour will surely be an ongoing trend. You can't turn on the television without seeing Eva Longoria, Sarah Jessica Parker, or some gorgeous celeb trying to sell you hair colour. TV and media will always have its place to sell more products but I believe as more women wake up and question why they are dying their hair and at what price, we will continue to see a shift towards natural beauty without all the use of chemicals.

In closing, I wanted to share a question I posed on social media to capture the divide on women going grey:

Question: If a study came out linking hair dye to breast cancer, would you stop dying your hair or take the risk? I am curious.

I received 136 comments. Here are some of my top picks to show you the divide on going grey:

- ✓ Sadly, probably not. I do take other precautions but that I could not cut out.
- ✓ I stopped having my hair coloured many years ago. I did not like the idea of all those chemicals soaking into my body.
- ✓ I think I would take the risk.
- ✓ I have not dyed my hair in ages, mostly a time issue, but yes, I would not dye if I was confident it was health risk.
- ✓ I started greying in my 20s. I would continue dying.
- ✓ Love this question. I would not dye my hair.
- ✓ Hmm, at this point in time, I'm sort of vain when it comes to my hair colour.
- ✓ I've already stopped! Authenticity & healthier!
- ✓ I don't die my hair. I decided in my twenties to just embrace the greys as they showed up.

✓ That would be very hard.

✓ No.

✓ I *am* stopping. I am so tired of going every five weeks; the expense, the dyes, the damage. I *do* like seeing myself, as I've always done, with dark hair, so the change will take time. I'm guessing it will look great when it's all grown in, so this is it, I'm taking the plunge.

✓ Hmm, I might look into wigs.

✓ Wow! I can't believe some think white or grey hair is worse than breast cancer.

✓ So many great natural products I'd try first if I wanted to dye it.

✓ I stopped long ago because I knew it was toxic!

✓ I don't like this question; I love hair colour.

✓ Don't ruin hair colouring for me, Nicole! Lol, but I guess I would look for a dye that didn't contain the ingredient that causes cancer.

✓ Add tattoo ink to the list of "colouring just for fun" while you are at it.

✓ That study has been out for years.

✓ This one got to me. Please add me to the group even though I don't have grey yet, I still highlight.

✓ I just wish I *had hair* to dye! (from a man … giggles)

✓ I'm embracing my grey as we speak.

✓ I would have a full head of white hair and I'm not 50. I would definitely try to seek a more natural dye if possible. But could not stop.

✓ I'm so glad I've stopped! Thanks for the support!

✓ I like my boobies and I think my hubby does too! Lol!

✓ I only highlight off the scalp so no dye touches my skin. But yes, if I did dye and breast cancer came up, I would ditch the dye. Plus, I love grey hair!

✓ Pls don't make me choose.

✓ I'm a breast-cancer survivor, and the first time I dyed my hair after it grew back in as grey, my friends went ballistic that I had dyed my hair. They were saying things like, "Don't you know that dye has toxic cancer-causing chemicals in it?" My answer was always appreciative for their concern, and I assured them that I was using a dye that was safe to use. I also mentioned that I had just been pumped through with every possible poison-filled chemical to kill my cancer, and save my life, and if it was the dye that caused me to go to my grave, I was going as a dark-haired person! Not all dyes are unsafe, and it's important to do your research on what to use. It is also a personal decision to make.

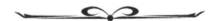

As you can see, this question brought out a big emotional divide. It is not an easy decision for most. We are caught between the influence of media and friends and deep-rooted ways of fitting in with society. It is a hot topic and is usually connected to a meaningful story that we created around going grey. I know I had to change my story. It took time. It took a health scare. It took deep reflection. It took bravery. Whatever your decision, may it be the best one for you.

CHAPTER THREE

What's Hiding in
Your Hair Dye?

"Don't let the noise of others' opinions drown out your own inner voice."

—STEVE JOBS

October 12, 2018, would be my last root touch-up forever. Let's go back to what happened that day. It was the usual quick in-and-out root touch-up. I felt the usual burn to the scalp, but this time I was more aware of the burn than ever. Why was it burning? What was in the dye that was causing me so much discomfort? Where in my body was that dye being absorbed? The toxic fumes filled my lungs with every breath I took, and I noticed a slight burn in my eyes. Even two days after my touch-up I was still feeling "off." My head was fuzzy and I had a headache, which I rarely ever get. My tongue had a toxic taste, which I've noticed before. This time was different though. I was tuned in. I was really paying attention to how I was feeling during and after my treatment. "Were those symptoms always there?" I asked myself. Did I really ignore them all those years of dyeing my hair? I was more aware than ever of my symptoms from the hair dye, and my inner voice was screaming at me, "Enough is enough, Nicole! You are smarter than this. You know your DNA weakness. You know that you are adding massive amounts of toxins to your body every three weeks, and you know that you have the power to control this. What if?" That was it. I made my decision right in that moment. No more. I was done with the root touch-up forever. That grey sparkle was going to come, and I was going to welcome it. I was doing this for my health. I was finally going to listen to my body.

Exposing the Ingredients

With my curious nature, I asked if I could take a picture of the ingredients list of my hair dye. Any guesses how many ingredients I was exposing my body to over the years? Over thirty! Holy crap! What about my hairdresser's health? I wonder how she feels after working with hair dye all week. How about all the hair dressers in the world, how does it impact them? Do they get sick more often? I wanted to know more about this industry and how hairdressers protected themselves from daily exposure.

As a holistic nutritionist, I teach families to read their food labels and avoid dyes in their food, and yet I was totally ignoring the label on my own hair dye. What the heck! I wondered how those chemicals on that list of ingredients could be impacting my health. The Environmental Working Group (EWG) has a cosmetics database that lists the hazards of each ingredient in a variety of products (see the resources section on page 235). For example, I learned that of the more than thirty ingredients in the product my hairdresser was using on me, over twenty of them were classified with effects ranging from "environmental toxin" to "skin irritant" to "immune and respiratory toxicant or allergen" to "human endocrine disruptor."[1]

"Endocrine disruptors," say what! The endocrine system is a network of glands that make hormones in your body that regulate metabolism, sexual function, sleep, mood, and much more. They include the thyroid, adrenal, ovaries, pancreas, and many other glands, and did you know that endocrine disruptors "may turn on, shut off, or modify signals that hormones carry? ... Some research suggests that these substances also adversely affect human health, ... resulting in reduced fertility and increased incidences or progression of some diseases, including obesity, diabetes, endometriosis, and some cancers."[2]

As you can see, the endocrine system is vital to our being able to achieve great health. Could all the toxins that I chose to ignore all those years have contributed to my estrogen-dominance symptoms? It's like playing a game of Russian roulette. I don't like playing that game, how about you? As I see it, reducing these toxins is an act of self-love, would you not agree?

How many friends do you have who suffer from these conditions? Do you think they are aware that the accumulation over the years of these toxins in their beauty products could be contributing to their health conditions today? I know it took my own health scare to wake me up and inspire me to rid my bathroom of these substances. Read your labels and dump the toxins!

The label on my hairdresser's hair dye also said, "Caution: Contains ammonia, 1-naphthol phenylenediamines (toluene diamines) resorcinol. Avoid eye contact. If eye contact occurs, rinse immediately. Wear suitable gloves. This product contains ingredients that can cause skin irritation/allergic reaction on certain individuals and a preliminary skin allergy test according to the accompanying direction should first be made 48 hours before each use. Keep out of reach of children. Hair colorants can cause severe allergic reactions."

The list of ingredients included names that I couldn't even pronounce. It looked like a chemical cocktail that only a scientist would understand. I immediately wanted to research every ingredient and learn more about what the warnings meant, such as what could a severe allergic reaction possibly look like? Have these ingredients been tested for safety? What kind of research has been done to protect consumers? Could these ingredients impact health? Could you actually die from your hair dye? What price are we prepared to pay for beauty? In my research I uncovered some of the side effects that we should consider before we become addicted to hair dye.

Side Effects of Hair Dyeing

The side effects of hair dyeing is a sensitive topic, and I understand because we are talking about limited and conflicting studies done in this area—and a billion-dollar industry that continues to grow. For decades, epidemiologists have been debating whether hair dye increases the risk of cancer. One of the problems is that there are large variations in the chemical content of hair dyes. This means that when a link is found, it is difficult to know which ingredient or chemical mix of ingredients is the culprit. In addition, cancer is a slow-developing disease in humans. By the time it surfaces, it is difficult to prove beyond a shadow of a doubt that one particular exposure was the cause. Who and what should we believe? It can be so confusing. Search Google and you will find information on both sides. Hair dye is safe. Hair dye can cause cancer. Hair dye is safe for pregnancy. Hair dye is not safe for pregnancy. My brain hurts digging into all this information, but I am committed to educating others on the health risks associated with hair dye.

Overprocessing

I witnessed my previous hairdresser go within a year from having gorgeous dark long curly healthy hair to overprocessed bleached blonde hair. What happened? She had the goal of platinum hair at age thirty. There was a big poster on the wall that showed a young model with platinum hair, and she wanted that. To go platinum she had to move from dark hair to white hair to have the grey colour adhere permanently. Unfortunately, she never made it without destroying her hair. She lost her hair in chunks, and in the end it was as dry and brittle as straw. "The constant hit of ammonia and peroxide over time damaged my hair," she said, "and I will never advise anyone to do what I did." Although processed hair can be revived to a certain extent with hair-care treatments, the only way to get rid of the damage from overprocessing is to chop your hair off. That is what she had to do. She stopped dyeing her hair, chopped it off, and had to begin the birth of a new head of hair. A big price to pay for overprocessed hair. I have found that with all my bleaching and lowlights, I have had to cut many inches off due to the damage from all these treatments. My new hairdresser recommended that we stop treating my hair with peroxide and lowlights or I risk losing chunks of hair and damaging it more. I am at a point now where I need to let the grey come in and be okay with a level of blending. It's not perfect. I see the skunk line, but my health is more important to me. I had a vision that when I started going grey I could have it blend in perfectly and no one would notice the transition. That has not been the case at all. I have had to accept that it's not perfect, and that's okay.

Allergies and Death

It isn't uncommon for hair dyes to cause allergic reactions, especially because permanent hair dyes contain paraphenylenediamine (PPD), which is a common allergen. People who have contact dermatitis are particularly prone to reactions because of the PPD and other chemicals present in dyes. People with skin conditions such as psoriasis and eczema should also refrain from using hair dyes to colour their hair. In milder cases, permanent dyes can cause burning, redness, itching, swelling, skin irritation, and blisters on your scalp or other sensitive areas such as your face and neck. Another thing to keep in mind when using these dyes is that not having had an allergic reaction in the past doesn't mean you won't have one in the future. There are many heartbreaking stories reported of people having severe reactions and even death due to hair dyes. I hadn't heard of this before, have you? Here were some of the headlines I found that hopefully will make you think twice before you use hair dye, or at least consider doing a patch test beforehand.

Headline #1

"Coroner Attacks Cosmetics Firms after Mother Died of Massive Allergic Reaction to Her L'Oréal Hair Dye"[3]

This article noted a woman who had slipped into a comma after using L'Oréal hair dye and never regained consciousness, and she died a year later.

Headline #2

"Hair Dye Ingredient Linked to Coma, Death"[4]

This article told of two teenage girls who claimed that their faces swelled up just days after using a semi-permanent colouring. Several weeks before this happened a seventeen-year-old died twenty minutes after she had dyed her hair. This article continued to highlight the concern around the colourant PPD in hair dye, and it also noted that Health Canada allows PPD in hair dye provided the label has clear warnings, but it has banned cosmetics with PPD that are applied directly to the skin. The article also noted a study published in the *Canadian Medical Association Journal* in 2007 that suggested that exposure PPD through products applied directly to the skin, even a small amount, could increase the likelihood of a reaction. The authors of this study reported that dermatologists are seeing increasing numbers of patients with allergic reactions to the PPD in black henna tattoos. The report concluded that this exposure to PPD results in "skin sensitization" to the chemical, resulting in subsequent exposure leading to a hypersensitivity.

As a side note, PPD is presently limited to 6% of the total hair dye content in the UK, but the chemical has been banned completely in Germany, France, and Sweden.[5]

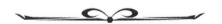

This was a big wake-up call for me. I had just come back from Mexico with nineteen family members, and a few of the younger nephews had received henna tattoos directly on their skin. We were lucky that none of them had a reaction. More than likely the tattoos had PPD as an ingredient, but at that time I wasn't thinking about the risk. Now that I am aware of this dangerous ingredient and the side effects, it will allow me to make different choices for my family and, hopefully, for yours too.

Asthma

Many studies[6,7,8] show that hairstylists who have a high exposure to hair dye are more susceptible to lung infections and developing asthma. Hair dyes aggravate asthma because of the persulphates present in them. Persulphates are chemicals found in bleaching agents, and hair dyes contain 60% of them. Asthma is often a consequence of constant exposure to PPD in hair dyes. Continued inhalation of persulphates can lead to throat discomfort, persistent cough, and asthma attacks.[9] Ammonia found in hair dyes may also contribute to asthma attacks. The exposure to these ingredients may sensitise your airway passages, making it difficult for you to breathe. Continued inhalation of these chemicals leads to throat discomfort, wheezing, lung inflammation, and coughing, as well as asthma attacks.

Cancer

When permanent hair dyes were first introduced, they contained chemicals, including some aromatic amines that were carcinogenic (cancer causing in mice). In 1976 one study reported that 87 of 100 breast cancer patients had been long-term hair dye users.[10] Although the formulas were later altered to replace these chemicals, the debate as to whether hair dyes can cause cancer remains controversial. Following are some studies that grabbed my attention:

1. In the early 1990s, Japanese and Scandinavian studies linked hair dye use with leukemia[11] and ovarian cancer.[12]

2. A 2001 study found that those who had worked for ten or more years as hairdressers or barbers had a fivefold risk of bladder cancer compared to the general population.[13]

3. An early Harvard study suggested that compared to women who had never dyed their hair, women who dyed their hair one to four times a year had a 70% increased risk for ovarian cancer.[14]

4. Researcher Sanna Heikkinen of the University of Helsinki, examined self-reported information from 8,000 Finnish women with breast cancer and a further 20,000 controls. She observed a 23% increase in breast cancer risk for those who regularly dyed their hair.[15]

5. In the hunt for the causes of breast cancer, researchers at the Rutgers Cancer Institute of New Jersey found two possible culprits: hair dye and relaxers, and more specifically, darker shades of hair dye.[16]

6. A review in 2013 found "alarming data" that pointed towards a link between hair-dye use in pregnancy and the development of several childhood malignancies in offspring. The authors recommended that "concerned pregnant women should avoid all hair colouring."[17]

7. A 2015 study published in *Occupational &
Environmental Medicine* linked the frequency of
dye and perm use to raised levels of carcinogens
found in hairdressers' blood.[18]

Some organizations caution against hair dyes, whereas
others say there isn't enough compelling evidence to be of
concern. Although some studies have linked the personal
use of hair dyes with increased risks of certain cancers of the
blood and bone marrow, such as non-Hodgkin lymphoma
(NHL) and leukemia, other studies have not shown such
links. Studies of bladder and breast cancer have also pro-
duced conflicting results. Relatively few studies have been
published about the association of hair dye use with the risk
of other cancers. Based on its review of the evidence, the International Agency for Research on Cancer Working Group
(IARC) concluded that the personal use of hair dyes is "not
classifiable as to its carcinogenicity to humans"[19] (although
they classify workplace exposure to hairdressers and barbers
is "probably carcinogenic to humans."[20] The National Toxicology Program (NTP) has not classified exposure to hair
dyes as to its potential to cause cancer. However, it has classified some chemicals that are or were used in hair dyes as
"reasonably anticipated to be human carcinogens."[21]

Here are my thoughts on this controversial topic. If we
all stopped dying our hair tomorrow for our health, the billion-dollar hair industry would come crashing down fast.
They would have to scramble to reinvent themselves to our
new standards of beauty and health. We know that will never happen. Why? Because we the consumers have bought
into the "look-good, feel-good" message that the media have
instilled in us over the last century. Until consumers stop
buying into these false messages of how we define beauty,

companies will continue to collect our money. However, small wins are happening that are challenging the norm. A big shoutout to Dove, which sought to change the culture of advertising by challenging beauty stereotypes and using real women to show true beauty, wrinkles and all. We have a long way to go, but small change is good because it can start a movement. So, as consumers we need to take a stand and decide what makes sense for us. What makes sense for you? What does your *gut* say? My momma-bear instinct says ditch the dye and let your *natural sparkle shine*!

Warning Labels

Given the history of consumers being harmed by hair dye over the years, the reason why there are warnings on your hair-dye packaging now makes sense. Let's review the common warnings on hair-dye products:

Warning #1

Do a skin test forty-eight hours before each use. I have never done a skin test with a salon or at home. Have you? What salon actually does this test? Who does a patch test at home? It sure seems that we are taking a big chance when we don't take a patch test. Please read the warnings on packages and do a skin patch test, it could save your life.

Warning #2

Wear suitable gloves. Why is this important? Poison control explains: "Gloves should be worn to limit the skin toxicity of hair dye. Many research studies have evaluated the use of gloves to reduce skin reactions from hair dyes, especially from dyes that contain PPD. One study found that nitrile gloves clearly outperform natural rubber latex, polyethylene, and vinyl gloves. Disposable gloves should never be re-used. Wearing gloves does not protect the scalp, neck, forehead, ears, and eyelids."[22]

If we protect our hands from the chemicals, how do you protect the skin on your head? I have had many hairdressers who never wear gloves, and they always have stained hands. That means they are playing in a chemical cocktail all day, which seems risky to me. Hairdressers, please wear your gloves. Home users, please wear your gloves.

Warning #3

"This product must not be used for dyeing eyelashes or eyebrows. To do so many cause blindness." Has anyone ever gone blind before from hair dye? Yes, they have. In England, a sixteen-year-old schoolgirl was blinded after suffering a severe allergic reaction to hair dye. The treatment at the hairdressers left her with blisters on her face and she was unable to open her eyes for five days. Now 21, she warns others about applying hair dye without completing a skin patch test beforehand.[23]

What Does the National Capital Poison Center (2016) Say about the Warnings?

"Even when hair dyes are used correctly, they can cause toxicity. Skin damage and allergic reactions are well documented. Eye exposure can cause a range of toxicities from mild irritation to loss of vision. Unintentional swallowing can cause irritation or injury to the mouth and stomach as well as life-threatening allergic reactions."[24]

What Does L'Oréal Say about This?

A spokeswoman for L'Oréal told the Brent and Kilburn Times: "Allergic reactions to hair colourants are extremely rare."[25] The spokeswoman also said that the allergy alert test must be completed before each colour application, even if you have previously used the same hair colourant or that of any other brand. "If you have ever experienced any reaction after colouring your hair or any reaction after temporary tattooing with black henna you should not proceed," she concluded.

I wonder how many women and men suffer symptoms but, like me, never report it. I accepted the scalp burn for years because of vanity. When I did use a more natural hair dye, I didn't get the burn, but the grey coverage wasn't as good, so I didn't use it as often and sometimes reluctantly went back to the chemical-laden home dyes. I'll discuss this further in chapter four, when we explore natural alternatives to dyeing your hair.

Food Colouring vs. Hair Colouring

The topic of food colouring as well as hair colouring is near and dear to my heart on many levels. As I mentioned earlier, my first career, for ten years, was in the food industry. When my daughter was diagnosed at nine months with food allergies, we had to stay away from all forms of chemicals, including food colouring. When I started to research food colouring and the link to cancer and behavioural issues in children, I was shocked! How could we allow these food additives into our food supply? How could we be okay adding them to children's foods? Was this money-motivated or health-motivated? I could write an entire book about what is happening to our food supply because it gets me fired up. The title of it would be *What the F*** Happened to our Food Supply and How Did We Let Them Get Away with It?* My point about food colouring is that they have been linked to cancer, organ damage, birth defects, and behavioural changes, and yet they are still allowed in our food supply. More and more parents are no longer okay with purchasing food that has food colouring as ingredients because they are becoming more aware of their effects on health, as I have listed below. We consumers have found our voices and are demanding better from companies more today than ever before.

Food Dyes and Their Effects[26]

Blue no. 1	Kidney tumours in mice and a possible effect on nerve cells
Blue no. 2	Tumours and brain gliomas
Citrus red no. 2	Toxic to rodents and tumours in urinary bladder
Green no. 3	Increases bladder cancer and testes tumour in rats
Red no. 3	Thyroid carcinogen in animals
Red no. 40 (most popular)	Tumours in mice
Yellow no. 5	Cancer-causing chemicals
Yellow no. 6	Adrenal tumors, cancer-causing chemicals

I personally witnessed my own daughter lose control of her behaviour and her body when she was exposed to food colourings. Her common symptoms were temper tantrums, inappropriate behaviour, hurting others, hyperactivity, and lack of focus. In my nutritional practice, I focused on helping families to clean up their diet and remove food colouring. Time and time again, parents were shocked to learn how this one simple change made such a huge impact to their children's mental health, their behaviour, and their happiness factor. So, if food colouring can have this much impact on our brain function, how about hair dye? It has colouring agents in it too!

People are speaking out about having chemical food colouring banned and shifting to natural food colouring,[27] but with little progress in North America. The British government forced businesses to stop using food dyes because they feared the health risk. What makes me angry as a mom is that you can get a healthier version of a candy bar in Europe (no chemical colours), and in North America we are still filled with toxic colours. For instance, Nestlé's chocolate "Smarties" in Europe contain radish, lemon, and red cabbage extracts for colouring rather than yellow no. 6 or red no. 40.[28] My least favourite holiday is Halloween as this is when the worst candy comes out and our kids get hammered with toxins. Ask a teacher what it's like the day after Halloween in the classroom. It's not pretty.

Seems as though Europe is ahead of the game when it comes to reduced chemicals in their food supply, and this is so even in their hair dye. The EU has banned or restricted over two thousand toxic ingredients that the US hasn't.[29] Canada's system of testing and regulating cosmetics is much more advanced than that of the United States, but there is still room for improvement. Health Canada has banned or restricted the use of over five hundred chemical ingredients for use in cosmetic products.[30] A list of these chemicals can be found on Canada's "Cosmetic Ingredient Hotlist," (see the resources section on page 235). Comparatively, the US has banned only eight chemical ingredients for use in cosmetics.[31]

Some companies are starting to wake up and remove some of the toxic chemicals, but we have a long way to go. What does this mean? How does it relate to hair dye? you might ask. Change takes time. When we are asking billion-dollar industries such as the food and hair industries to make change for the "health of it" without impacting their bottom line, change is slow. Why use chemicals? They're cheaper, they're brighter, they're more stable, and also because sometimes the naturally coloured products aren't as bright as the synthetically coloured ones, and so they're not as attractive to consumers. We have a long way to go, not only to clean up our food supply, but our beauty products as well. For now, my advice to you, my readers is to read your labels, choose wisely, and listen to your gut feelings. The great news is that more and more healthier alternatives are coming out, giving us healthier options for food and beauty products. Your buying behaviour sends a message to companies. You are the ones who make change. You are the ones who say "we want fewer chemicals in our products." Next time you buy a product at the grocery store, ask yourself, "Is my purchase sending the right message back to this company?"

What Types of Toxins Are Found in Hair Dye?

Too many. The National Cancer Institute (NCI) states that over 5,000 different chemicals are used in hair-dye products. The Environmental Working Group has ranked over 450 hair colours in their Skin Deep Cosmetics Database (see the resources section on page 235), and roughly 400 of them are considered a high hazard because they contain toxins linked to cancer; allergies; and irritation of the eyes, skin, or lungs; immunotoxicity and organ toxicity; developmental and reproductive toxicity; and neurotoxicity. More specifically, on the box of your hair-dye product at home, or in the dyes used at your salon, you may find the following toxic ingredients:

- Para-phenylenediamine and tetrahydro-6-nitroquinoxaline: Both of these have been shown to damage genetic material and cause cancer in animals
- Methylparaben: Cause endocrine disruption and allergies/immunotoxicity
- Ammonia: A chemical that can irritate the skin, nose, throat, respiratory system, and eyes
- Peroxide: Can cause serious skin, eye, and lung irritation; immunotoxicity; and allergies
- Eugenol: A fragrance ingredient that's associated with cancer, immunotoxicity, neurotoxicity, and allergies
- Coal tar: A known carcinogen
- Lead acetate: Possible link between this chemical and fertility issues in men and women. For years this toxin has been banned in the European Union and in Canada. The US announced in 2018 that they will also ban this toxin from all cosmetics
- Formaldehyde: A preservative linked to cancer, developmental and reproductive toxicity, and more

Of course, these are just a few common toxic ingredients in hair dye today. As mentioned at the beginning of this chapter, the hair dye at the salon I went to contained over thirty ingredients, each of which I researched to learn of their possible side effects. This exercise was alarming to me. If you have a box of hair colour under your bathroom sink, I encourage you to look up some of the ingredients for yourself using the Skin Deep Cosmetics Database. The results may just shock you!

Is It Safe for Your Kids to Dye Their Hair?

My momma instinct would say *no*, it is not safe. Kids Colouring their hair at an earlier age just adds more toxins to their growing bodies. Our kids are growing up in a much more toxic world than we did. A review of scientific reports[32] noted that –

1. "The European Chemicals Agency estimates there are more than 144,000 man-made chemicals in existence. The US Department of Health estimates 2000 new chemicals are being released every year. The UN Environment Program warns most of these have never been screened for human health safety."

2. "The World Health Organization estimates that 12 million people—one in 4—die every year from diseases caused by 'air, water and soil pollution, chemical exposures, climate change and ultraviolet radiation,' all of which result from human activity."

There are many chemicals that a child could potentially absorb or have an adverse reaction to. Dr. Sejal Shah, MD, a New York–based dermatological surgeon, advises against hair-dye use in children. "I really don't think it's safe to dye or bleach a child's hair until after puberty, and ideally not until their late teens—at least 16."[32] Kids' hair is much finer and their skin more sensitive, so they are more likely to experience reactions. If you decide to dye your child's hair make sure to do a 48-hour patch test.

The weight of the evidence, clearly suggests a need for caution. Looking at both sides, I have to believe hair dye is risky, especially when used frequently and with dark colours. "Risky" you ask. What other risky habits in our lives do we have that we don't think twice about, such as drinking alcohol, smoking, eating processed food, eating vegetables sprayed with pesticides, eating too much sugar, not moving enough physically, and lathering our bodies daily with chemical-laden beauty products. Where do we draw the line? Do we choose to live in a bubble? We'll never live a life free of toxins, and that's okay because our bodies are designed to handle a certain amount of exposure. Our goal should be to prioritize our exposures to stay as healthy as possible, while still enjoying life! I am glad I ditched the dye—it made sense for me. Maybe it doesn't make sense to you right now and you're looking for healthier alternatives. Join me in the next chapter, where I showcase healthier options for people not ready to ditch the dye.

CHAPTER FOUR

Healthier Options if You're Not Ready to Go Grey

"To be beautiful means to be yourself. You don't need to be accepted by others. You need to accept yourself."

—Author unknown

At thirty-five, thirteen years ago, I had enough grey hair that it was becoming annoying. That little voice of fear inside of me was whispering in my ear, "You are not ready to go grey, Nicole." Can you relate? From everything I had learned when I was studying to be a nutritionist, I knew I should stop dying my hair, but I'm not going to lie, vanity trumped. Month after month I kept dying my hair, ignoring the health consequences.

Whatever your age, and you are dying your hair to cover the grey, I don't judge you. But I care about your health, which is why I'm writing this chapter. This chapter is about how we can still cover our grey hair, but with a reduced chemical hit to our bodies.

I have researched healthier options from around the world to share with you here—stories from hairstylists and friends and companies that provide chemical-free solutions to dying your hair.

Are There Hair Salons that Use Organic, Clean Products?

The answer to this is yes. I want to introduce you to three hair-salon owners who care deeply about their mission to provide natural care for their clients. I share their stories with you here and introduce you to the products they choose to use.

1. *Energy Organic Salon, Newmarket, Ontario, Canada*[1]
Owner: Kristina Iacovides
Mission: Energy Organic Salon recognizes that health and beauty go hand in hand. The products that you use on your skin and in your hair are just as important as the food you eat. Therefore, we choose to offer natural and organic products that promote a healthy lifestyle.

Kristina is the owner and master stylist of Energy Organic Salon as well as a registered holistic nutritionist. With over eighteen years of experience in the hair industry, Kristina specializes in a variety of styles, colour techniques, and cutting variations. She started when she was seventeen years old when she came across a newspaper ad that caught her attention and subsequently launched her into a new career. She worked for fifteen years in Newmarket at various salons and was exposed for forty hours a week to toxic chemicals without realizing their impact on her own health.

Kristina began her journey in the fitness and holistic health world over eight years ago. Having dealt with her own challenges of severe allergies, weight gain, sleep problems, hormones, and liver issues, she was determined to heal her body. Kristina decided to take matters into her own hands and researched and studied holistic health to improve her own life. Having seen the incredible results and benefits that came with those life changes, Kristina felt compelled to share this knowledge. Influenced by her own health challenges, her new-found knowledge of nutrition, and having her mom and aunt both experience cancer, she had a vision of owning an organic salon one day. She wanted to create a safe environment for herself, her staff, and her clients that was affordable for everyone. Her vision became a reality and Energy Organic opened in 2016.

Kristina is strongly committed to improving the health and welfare of her clients and people in the community. She has done volunteer work for cancer and mental-health fundraisers and has worked with low-income families. As she says, "I am excited to now amalgamate my two worlds of hair styling and holistic health. I care deeply about my clients and not only want to take care of their hair needs but I am proud to also offer them a better service for their health."

Kristina shopped the world before she decided to support two hair-product lines that met her high standards of being toxin free:

- Organic Colour Systems, UK
- O&M (Original & Mineral), Australia

I thank Kristina for being brave and taking a risk. She has a beautiful salon that allows women and men to dye their hair safely without harsh chemicals. She is truly making a difference in her community.

(See the resources section on page 235 for Energy Organic Salon's website.)

2. *Green Hair Zone, Newmarket, Ontario, Canada*[2]

Owner: Lana Demkovic

Lana Demkovic is the owner of the organic hair salon, Green Hair Zone, and has been a top professional hair stylist for almost two decades. Lana possesses extensive knowledge in various cutting and texturizing techniques, and she is an expert in mixing colour for all stages of the application.

Her journey to opening a healthier salon without harsh chemicals started during her first pregnancy. She couldn't work while pregnant in her regular salon without feeling sick. The same thing happened with her second pregnancy, and those experiences planted a seed for her. Over time, she started noticing that she would go home with headaches and feeling tired, and the chemical smells began to bother her more and more. She started researching healthier ways to dye hair and got excited about the possibility of offering better solutions for her clients. Four years ago, she made the move and opened up her own organic salon for the sake of her own health and that of her clients.

What she didn't expect after opening her salon was the number of women who started sharing their past experiences of using toxic chemicals. She was shocked at how many women had symptoms of burning scalp, rashes, and headaches every time they dyed their hair, but they never said anything. Once she opened her salon and started using her Organic Colour Systems product line, she was so excited that she was getting great hair results without the use of harsh chemicals. Her customers felt happier for not experiencing anymore unhealthy side effects. Lana said, "Women didn't really talk about their symptoms from the dyes, they just sucked it up and figured that this was the price you pay to look good." Now with her new salon and healthier products, more and more of her clients are realizing there is a better way. Lana told me she figures about 50% of her clients were having unhealthy symptoms from chemical dyes, and now she is happy to report that they are symptom-free since changing over to the organic product line. She shopped North America and tested many products before making her final selection with Organic Colour Systems. It is more expensive, she said, but it works great and clients love how they feel.

Lana's Green Commitment: We are committed to "Reducing our carbon footprint" not only by using organic hair products but also by lowering our energy consumption.

Our salon was purposely designed and built to reduce energy waste as much as possible. Our mechanical systems are all energy efficient: HVAC, hot water tank, washer, and dryer. The lighting was designed and built with LED-powered fixtures. The emergency lighting is LED system as well.

We have reused materials throughout the entire construction, forming, back framing, and so on. The reception desk and long corridor bench were built from leftover structural wood and steel. All the walls are well insulated and the precast walls come with insulation built inside the panels.

The concrete waste was recycled and the excavated soil repurposed. We are proud to say that after all construction, we sent only two construction vans with excess materials to garbage collection. We have incorporated existing building features: concrete walls, structural steel into our design, and avoided to waste more construction materials. Porcelain, glass and stone tiles used are recyclable products as well. Our salon was painted with 0% VOC paint from Sherwin Williams. At Green Hair Zone, they say, "We love what we do, and this is our way of giving back to our clients, community, and earth."

I thank Lana for introducing me to safer products to support my transition to my natural hair colour. It was so wonderful to find a salon where my symptoms from toxins, such as headaches, scalp burning, and a toxic taste on my tongue vanished after using their healthy products. She is making such a difference in her community.

(See the resources section on page 235 for Green Hair Zone's website.)

3. Henna Hair Salon, Whitby, Ontario, Canada[3]
Owner: Gina Laurito

Gina's hairstylist career started when she was nineteen years old. She spent ten years as a traditional hairdresser working daily with chemicals. As her health started to decline in those early years, she began to question the toxins in her salon environment. Could these toxins be contributing to her poor health? She was curious. She suffered from chronic bladder infections that would often travel to her kidneys, and she was prescribed one antibiotic after another. On top of that she had chronic sinus infections, so she couldn't ignore her poor health any longer. She was too young to be sick all the time, and she was motivated to feel well again. She started to listen to the inner nudge and got the message that she needed to make a change for the better. She sold her traditional salon in one month and spent six months on a healing journey. She detoxed her body, and her symptoms disappeared and haven't returned since she left that toxic salon environment. Gina dove into researching the dangers of hair dye and alternative options for a chemical-free experience. She knew she wanted to work with henna after she realized it had many health benefits while still offering great results for the hair. Her dream for a chemical-free salon came true when she opened up her first location in 2009. Gina's health has never been better and she feels so good to be offering chemical-free solutions to her clients.

I thank Gina for bringing such a unique toxin-free plant-based hair salon to our community. My hope is for more of these hair salons to pop up all over the world.

(See the resources section on page 235 for Henna Hair Salon's website.)

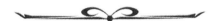

As you have read, all three hairstylists changed their work environment and the products they used to gain better health for themselves and their clients. They took a chance. They risked the unknown and it worked for them. They have thriving businesses and have found a niche in the marketplace. They are healthier and happier because of the changes they made. Their change became their new passion and mission to contribute to a healthier world. Well done, ladies, you have inspired me with your stories. Now let's take a look at some hair and beauty companies that took a risk and developed healthier products.

Organic Colour Systems, UK[4]

Organic Colour Systems' journey started over two decades ago with one very clear mission: To provide hairdressers with a less toxic and more natural-based range of colours, care, and styling options. Established in 1994, Organic Colour Systems became industry pioneers in the introduction of natural and organic-based products to the salon professional market. The managing director, Raoul Perfitt, has a background in herbal medicine. His grandfather was the forefather of the herbal-medicine movement in the UK. Raoul also had a friend, Stephen, who was severely allergic to hair colour. Stephen was a hairdresser and didn't want to give up the career he passionately loved, so he and Raoul came up with the concept that resulted in the Organic Colour Systems.

So, what is the meaning behind their name? When Organic Colour Systems was established, their name was determined by two key influences: (1) A promise to use the most natural ingredients possible in all of their products and minimize the harsh use of chemicals. They use synthetic ingredients only where a suitable organic or natural alternative is not available. (2) The *Oxford English Dictionary* defines "organic" as "of the elements of a whole, harmoniously related." Organic Colour Systems is a system. Their product range was developed to work in synergy as a whole. All elements of the range of products work in harmony to give the best professional results and keep the hair in optimum condition. They champion an organic lifestyle and the health benefits that this way of life brings, not only to individuals but also to the eco-system on which we all rely.

Organic Colour Systems does use PPD in some of their hair-colour products because it is required to achieve a true black. Although PPD is known to produce allergic reactions, 99.9% of permanent oxidative hair colours contain PPD (or PTD or PTS), the main pigments used in mainstream hair-colour products. However, Organic Colour Systems uses the lowest level off PPD possible, averaging 0.36% compared to the EU maximum legal limit of 4% at concentrate. Even so, Organic Colour Systems always recommend skin sensitivity tests.

Organic Colour Systems also uses ethanolamine (MEA), an ammonia-free ingredient that raises the pH of the hair, which is required for the colour to take hold. Ammonia is known for its production of irritating gas, but MEA can also have negative side effects on the hair. However, the base colour is already alkaline so it raises the pH of the hair so far less MEA is required.

Organic Colour Systems feels privileged to have a like-minded community of professional stylists in thousands of salons, in over forty countries across the globe. Today, Organic Colour Systems is striving to make hairdressing a healthier industry worldwide.

(See the resources section on page 235 for Organic Colour Systems' website.)

O&M, Australian Born Hair Care⁵

The Original & Mineral Journey: Pioneering Clean Colour and Natural Luxury

O&M's vision is to bring nature and luxury together in a line of Australian born hair colour, care and styling products that are safe, effective, and beautiful to use. Developed by a band of rule-breakers and pioneers, the brand's core values are a commitment to making the world safer and more beautiful—and having fun while they do it.

They challenge the artificial norms of professional haircare with formulations that are both effective and gentle, removing harsh chemicals wherever possible, while including Australian natural extracts and active minerals that deliver real benefits.

O&M founder and CEO Jose Bryce Smith says, "I have always been passionate about natural products, wellbeing, and beauty. When I saw first-hand how harsh chemical products affected hairdressers and clients, I knew that hair colour would eventually become a health choice. Originally, we just wanted a safer alternative for pregnant women, people with sensitivities and hairdressers breathing in chemicals every day. As O&M evolved, it became for everyone."

Jose's former partner, a hairdresser, suffered from contact dermatitis, making it impossible for him to use conventional hair colour. Together, they opened the first ammonia-free salon in Australia nearly two decades ago, which attracted a progressive clientele and gave Jose the confidence to take the O&M vision further.

In 2010, O&M Method, the care and styling line, was launched. Packaged luxuriously, these products had and still have a "Free from Five" formulation—no harmful sulphates, parabens, propylene glycol, MIT, or Triclosan. Now certified by PETA (People for the Ethical Treatment of Animals) as cruelty-free, today O&M Method is stocked in leading hair salons around the world, as well as high-end e-commerce and retail destinations, including Sephora USA and Southeast Asia, NET-A-Porter, and adorebeauty.com.au.

As the world changes, and low-chemical and natural technology is becoming mainstream, O&M continues to lead the way. In 2013, they did what many chemists said was impossible, when they developed Clean Colour Technology—permanent professional hair colour with zero ammonia, PPD, or resorcinol. It was a ground breaker that performed with no smell or fumes while giving results to match conventional hair colour.

Then, in 2017, with the help of world-leading chemists, O&M evolved again. On a mission to provide the cleanest professional colour in the world, O&M discovered a progressive new colouring approach: Molecular Blend Technology. In MBT, pre-linked colour pigments supported by two nourishing hero complexes give incredible vibrancy, shine, longevity, and protection. This new generation of low-chemical high-performance colour is called O&M CØR.color.

As the Ø in the name suggests, CØR.color is true to O&M's core promise: zero ammonia, PPD, or Resorcinol. Original & Mineral is a complete salon solution, made for hairdressers by hairdressers.

(See the resources section on page 235 for O&M's website.)

Herbatint, retail product available in over forty countries[6]
Herbatint was the product my mom found when she started working in a health-food store in the 1990s. I saw her using it for years, covering up her grey hair with success. When I went back to school and became a nutritionist, this was the brand I started to use at home.

Herbatint's Story
Herbatint, the main brand of the Italian Antica Erboristeria, was developed in 1970 by herbalist Michele Albergo. In the 1060s, Mr. Albergo also founded Antica Erboristeria, a company that specializes in ammonia-free permanent hair colour based on herbal extracts. In creating Herbatint, he focused his research on finding the gentlest possible formulation for effective hair colour at a time when the industry was dominated by multinationals whose products were based heavily on ammonia and other harsh chemicals.

Michele Albergo was strongly influenced by a Swiss herbalist with whom he'd carried out his apprenticeship as a young man. This master herbalist quickly came to appreciate the passionate young Italian who assisted him in developing his herb-based cosmetics, and upon his death, having no heir, he left Mr. Albergo in possession of his entire collection of research and formulas, some of which had been handed down through his family from generation to generation.

That was the beginning of Mr. Albergo's long quest to find that perfect synergy between herbal extracts that would offer the most natural alternative to chemical hair dyes. By the end of the sixties, Mr. Albergo had created a formula for a permanent hair dye based on plant extracts with a very low percentage of hydrogen peroxide and no ammonia. This extraordinary formula assured perfect coverage of grey hair from its first application, without damaging the hair while delivering natural shades. Herbatint was born!

Forty years on, Herbatint has been the undisputed market leader, gaining a well-deserved reputation and now being sold in more than forty countries.

(See the resources section on page 235 for Herbatint's website.)

The Green Beaver Company (Canadian Born)

Since our launch in 2002, Green Beaver has sought to provide healthy, natural products for your family and for ours. Founded by husband-and-wife team Karen Clark and Alain Ménard, whose work in the pesticide and pharmaceutical industries helped shape their interest in natural goods, Green Beaver was developed as a reaction to the harsh chemicals found in children's shampoos, bubble baths, and other self-care products.

After years of working as biochemists and microbiologists, Karen and Alain were appalled at the amount of dangerous ingredients used to create hygiene products, especially for children. So much so that Karen left her job in 1995 to begin formulating products that would eventually become Green Beaver mainstays. Additionally, it was when Alain's 32-year-old sister was diagnosed with breast cancer in 1999—a disease often linked to the parabens used in everyday products like deodorant—that Green Beaver truly became a team initiative.

The goal was simply to put their knowledge to better use and create a difference in the world by providing all-natural alternatives. In 2001, Karen and Alain welcomed their son, Joshua, into the family. He was the true inspiration for Green Beaver's launch – after all, Karen and Alain had set out to provide healthy options to future generations of Canadian families.

Between 2003 and 2009, Green Beaver thrived. Karen and Alain formulated new products, travelled to trade shows and health food stores, grew their brand, and put their energy into educating consumers about the benefits of all-natural ingredients. By the end of 2009, they became officially Ecocert certified and built their own production facility in Hawkesbury.

The spring of 2011 brought a big first for Canadians and Green Beaver alike: They launched the first Canadian organic mineral sunscreen with the help of the National Research Council. In the years to follow, they continued to launch products that would change the way Canadians and neighbouring countries would care for themselves and their families. They developed the Organic Honey Lip Balm to combat the precipitous decline of bees and developed soaps, deodorants, and toothpastes to better serve the growing community of natural skin care lovers.

Through better understanding of natural ingredients like sunflower oil, Labrador tea, lavender, and other organic elements, they made sustainable, reliable products with the environment and people in mind. In 2016, they became the *first Canadian company to be Plastic Microbead-free* since day one and their products were added to the Zero database.

Nowadays, after doubling their production line and continuing to educate consumers on the risks of chemicals, Green Beaver maintains its dedication to natural goodness. Regardless of their company's growth, they have always remained dedicated to using certified organic Canadian ingredients. They are still a family-owned company and just like the name suggests, Green Beaver is a truly natural and purely Canadian brand.

"We all have the power to change the industries that are causing harm, and we can do it simply by choosing what we consume." —Alain Ménard, Co-founder

(See the resources section on page 235 for The Green Beaver Company's website.)

Let's Talk Henna

Henna, also known as Mehndi in Hindi, has been used since antiquity in the Arabian Peninsula, the Indian subcontinent, the Near East and Middle East, and Northern Africa and the Horn of Africa to dye and decorate the skin, hair, and fingernails as a symbol of beauty.

The leaves of select plants are ground up, and when mixed with water the tannins in the plant produce a dye pigment that is similar to your hair protein, making it ideal for hair colour as well as for protecting, strengthening, and beautifying the hair. Henna is good for you and your hair, and you can apply it as often as you like. It also has antifungal and antibacterial properties, and it contains no toxic chemicals, it is environmentally friendly, and it is 100% natural. Henna also helps to treat dandruff, eczema, and dry scalp, and it promotes hair growth.

When used to colour your hair, you will find that with every henna application the colour deepens and becomes richer and you will experience beautiful hair. When I interviewed Gina at Henna Hair Salon, she said, "It only takes me twenty-five minutes to mix and apply henna to my clients' hair. Then, for best results, I wrap their hair and they go home and rinse it off a few hours later." So, yes, my friends, you will need to give yourself an afternoon or evening to be wrapped up with the henna, but the benefit is beautiful chemical-free hair.

Below is a list of the plants that Gina uses with her clients. She sources them from organic farms in India. You can go to her website to place an order and learn how to apply the henna and other plants at home if you can't make it to her salon in Whitby. (See the resources section on page 235.)

Plant	Effect
Henna	Gives reddish tones for brunettes and copper tones for white or fair hair
Indigo	Indigo on its own dyes hair a blue tone, and it neutralizes warm tones created by henna.
Cassia	This Ayurvedic herb will leave your hair glossy, stronger, thicker, dandruff-free, and healthy. *Cassia obovata* gives you all the benefits of henna without affecting the colour of on dark hair tones.
Amla berry	Gives a cool golden tone to henna mixtures and conditions the hair and boosts curl

Next up, a personal story from one of my mentors and dear friend, Dr. Mitra Ray. She recently shared her story with me about how she became very sick with PPD exposure and the impact it had on her health. Her story really hit my heart and she was kind enough to put into words her journey with PPD exposure and the chemical-free options she found to support her healthy lifestyle.

Dr. Mitra Ray's Biography

As a biochemist with a PhD in cellular biology from Stanford University, Dr. Ray worked in the arena of degenerative diseases, such as cancer and Alzheimer's disease. Her research was funded by the National Institutes of Health, the American Cancer Society, and an Alzheimer's research grant. In 1994, she made an important and personal discovery that radically changed her life and her work. She changed her diet, exercise routine, and lifestyle, and her back pain subsided. Preventive concepts in health, such as whole-food nutrition, became her new direction in research.

Dr. Mitra Ray's Story[8]

I just needed a haircut before going to an event where I was to speak. We were living in London, UK, at the time, and I was excited to find a cute little salon in the neighbourhood. The gal cutting my hair was good at making conversation, and she asked if I had noticed how much grey hair I had on the back of my head, which she also said was unusual as she didn't see much on the front. I felt my heart skip a beat. I was too embarrassed to admit to her that I often plucked out any grey strands I saw when I looked in the mirror, but I didn't pay much attention to what might be going on at the back of my head. It just never occurred to me that I also had grey hair where I couldn't see. I always felt that grey hair betrayed my youthfulness, and I felt that this was completely unacceptable. The hairdresser must have noticed my immediate change of mood, and she gently offered to colour my hair at a discount, right then and there.

I should have asked for a patch test instead of reacting to my own emotions.

Walking home, I felt so good with a fresh haircut and no grey anywhere. I felt more prepared for an event coming up, and now I had only to work on my speech. Later that evening my head began to itch, and it got progressively worse to the point where I barely slept that night. When I looked in the mirror at the first light of dawn, I saw that my eyes were red and swollen and my face had begun to swell up. I was in complete shock of what was happening. "Why me? What just happened?" is all I could think. When my husband and kids woke up and saw me, the look on their faces spoke volumes. That was just day one. As the days progressed, my face kept blowing up and the itching turned into burning pain. There was no relief and I felt as though I was going to lose my mind.

Why didn't I just go to the doctor or the hospital? Because I didn't feel safe doing that. I had recently lost my dad and I had blamed modern medicine for the loss. He was one data point in one giant and unregulated experiment, as he was one of the early recipients of the first generation of pace makers and defibrillators, not to mention a whole cabinet full of medications with some scary side effects. I was still too raw from loss of my father. Going to a doctor in a London was just not an option in my mind. Maybe if I had been back at home in Seattle, I would have made a different choice.

I also felt ridiculously stupid that, as a biochemist, I hadn't been patient and done a patch test, that I hadn't ever heard about PPD allergies before this incident, and that I was now the victim of all this ignorance. I was in so much pain and agony, and it had all been avoidable.

To fast forward, it took over four weeks for the itching, burning, and extreme swelling to calm down. And then my skin had stretched so much that I looked like I was ninety years old. It took an entire year and a few cleanses for me to look my age again. As someone who made their living promoting health and nutrition, I had to go into hiding during this entire time as no one would have taken my advice given the way I looked.

This had happened in 2006, but it would not be my last exposure. Several years later, I was given the gift of a facial, and I felt it would be impolite to not accept. While I had a towel over my eyes, the aesthetician noticed that I had grey hairs in my eyebrows, and she recommended this natural dye from Germany that she thought would help me. I calmly told her of my dye allergies, but she insisted that this was all natural and proceeded to apply it to my eyebrows. I thought she was applying an innocuous cream, but then she told me that she had died my eyebrows. I sat up in shock. She saw my expression and quickly said that it was complimentary and apologized. Well the money and the apology were not going to save me from a second exposure, and another round of a nightmare reaction. Once again I was mad at myself, mad at the ignorance of beauticians and aestheticians, mad that there was such a chemical called PPD that was allowed to be in dyes, and mad that I had fallen prey one more time! Was there a lesson here for me to learn?

Since I am solution oriented, I began to look into henna and became quite versed in what works and what does not work. I do know that you cannot be tripped up by henna products with any additives or formulations. There is no shortcut to using henna. I recommend the two-step method of pure *Lawsonia inermis* (henna) powder and *Indigofera tinctoria* (indigo) powder. You have to make up the henna powder twelve to twenty-four hours in advance to freshly shampooed hair and leave it on for at least thirty minutes, and then apply the pure indigo mix, which should be made forty-five minutes in advance of application. Any method that tries to combine the two steps doesn't work well. (See the resources section on page 235 for the instructions, in particular chapter 7, "Mixing and Testing Your Henna Mix.")

Why does it have to be pure henna powder (*Lawsonia inermis*) and indigo powder (*Indigofera tinctoria*)? Well that takes me to my third and final exposure. I was in India a few years ago and my cousin's wife, who is my age, was raving about how she had found a great henna that worked really well. Given how hard it is to make the henna work right, I was intrigued. I was rushing to get ready to leave for the airport to get my daughter when my cousin's wife said, "Hey, before you shower and go, I just made up some henna so let me quickly apply it and you can see how well it works." I was in such a rush that I didn't think it through. I was excited to see my daughter who had been travelling the world on a global studies program, and I was in India, the land of henna, and so my defenses were naturally down. So I let her put the henna in, then I quickly showered and headed to the airport. Well, during the car ride there my scalp started to itch! I called while driving to have my cousin's wife send me a picture of the label, and sure enough, PPD was in the mix. How stupid was I? This time I decided I would take drugs because there was no way I was going through all that pain and agony again. However, I couldn't find a doctor in India who would give me anything stronger than Benadryl or Claritin. A week later, I had a nightmarish flight back to Seattle, and once I landed, I finally got a prescription for prednisone. Although it did calm down the hellish reaction, prednisone is not a fun drug to be taking. It took several months and several doctors until I finally found someone who could help me properly wean me off the prednisone without my body having a ghost reaction to the PPD.

So, I have had three rounds of reactions to PPD. It may seem that I am a total idiot and perhaps that vanity and stupidity are the cause of my suffering. However, I will tell you this. PPD is the cause of my suffering. I have spent over thirty-five years studying health as a research scientist and as a promoter of alternative or integrative modalities of healing. I live a fairly clean life and am super conscious of the food I put in my mouth as well as the products we have in the house for cleaning ourselves and our house. I have written books on health and have run health retreats for decades. I am not ignorant nor particularly vain. In fact, if I had mostly grey hair, I would just go grey. I have just enough that it is annoying and not a great look that would make me feel good to go *tout naturel*. I have seen many hairdressers to whom I tried to explain my situation, and I have received very little sympathy or recognition that there even is a problem with hair dyes.

One explanation for PPD sensitivity is that about one in two hundred people have large pores in their scalp, and PPD can enter through the scalp, and into the blood stream, which causes the extreme immune response/severe allergy.

Also, because our bodies do change over time, anyone can become PPD sensitive over time. There are some alternative hair dyes that are being sold with PPD derivatives, but they are also dangerous to those who are PPD sensitive. Before any application, always, always do a patch test to see what your sensitivity level is.

It's stories like Dr. Mitra Ray's that hopefully make us think twice before we say yes to the dye. The world is changing fast. More and more people are demanding toxin-free products and companies are listening. Henna would be my first choice, just as it is for Dr. Ray. If you're not ready to go grey, and henna seems like too much work, here is a short list of cleaner hair products to consider, just be cautious of the level of PPD in the formula if you are sensitive.

Hair Colour Products[9]
Herbatint Permanent Haircolor Gel
Naturtint Permanent Hair Color
Tints of Nature Permanent Hair Color
Light Mountain Natural Hair Color & Conditioner
Logona Natural Herbal Botanical Hair Color
Surya Brasil Henna Hair Cream
Naturigin Permanent Hair Color
Madison Reed Root Touch Up
Radico Colour Me Organic Hair Color
O&M Mineral CCT Permanent Hair Color

So, you're still not ready to go dye free? No problem. My hope is that this chapter inspired you enough to look at what you are using to dye your hair and to consider a healthier option. You might also consider the following:

Do you have symptoms every time you dye your hair, as I did?

- Are you ignoring them, as I did?
- Will you consider a patch test to avoid the risk of a severe reaction?
- Will you try henna?
- Will you seek out an organic salon?
- Will you buy healthier products?
- Will you let your kids dye their hair often because it's cool?

Whatever you decide to choose, do it wisely! We live in a world where we are exposed daily to toxins. Some we can control and some we cannot. We know that over time those toxins can build up in our bodies and make us sick if we don't pay attention. The good news is that we can control what we put on our hair and skin. Thank you to the brave hairstylists and companies that are paving the way to a healthier way to take care of our hair.

CHAPTER FIVE

Our Biggest Fears
of Going Grey

"Our deepest fear is not that we are inadequate. Our deepest fear is that we are powerful beyond measure."
—MARIANNE WILLIAMSON

What does fear have to do with going grey? Everything. Let's dive in to see what and where this fear comes from. When my sister planted that seed about going grey, I immediately started having a boxing match in my head. I wish I could have recorded the conversation I had with myself. I'm sure it was entertaining. It's amazing the mind games you start playing with yourself when an idea shows up that scares you. You start justifying why not to do something, and I was witnessing it right in front of me. I was having a secret conversation with myself, saying, "You're only forty-seven years old, Nicole. You work in the wellness industry and you have to look young and vibrant. Grey hair will age you fast. You're just out of a twenty-year marriage and you need to look hot and sexy." On and on these stories played in my head until I convinced myself that grey hair was not for me.

My sister and I started talking about when our mom decided to grow her grey hair out before she hit fifty, and how we had not been supportive. What was it that we didn't support? We soon realized that it was fear. Fear that by looking older, our mom would begin to play the part of an older person and be less capable of participating in life. For a young adult, that is a scary thing to contemplate— your parents getting old. It really does bring out fear. The reality that your parents won't be around forever, and the grey is just another thing that reminds us of our deepest fear, losing the ones we love. I am actually welling up with tears as I write this because I can't imagine my life without my parents. They have been my rock. So now I understand when my teenage girls are resisting my grey movement. It now makes sense. All I needed to do was go back to when my mom announced her decision and realize that I had not been happy either. The only role models I had in my life when my mom announced that she was going grey were my grandparents. My closest grandma was not only grey, but she also seemed to be old and frail. That vision of an old, frail grandma was my fear of where my mom was headed. That was terrifying.

My mom never did follow my grandma's path. She made major changes over the years, which included no more drinking, no more dyeing, and maintaining an active and healthy lifestyle. I recently went down to Ecuador to visit my mom, and everyone asked if we were sisters. I hope I look as good as my mom does now in her mid-sixties.

My mom has become a role model for me. Not only for her passion to embrace a healthy lifestyle, but also her standing in her power of aging gracefully and beautifully. I was determined to achieve optimal health more than anything, and that meant grey was going to have to be part of my new normal. Yes, it may make me look older. Yes, it may wash my face out. Yes, it will generate a lot of talk, but who cares? I was done. I wanted a healthy body and was willing to do whatever it takes.

A day in October 2018 was such an *empowering* moment for me when I made the decision to stop dyeing my roots. The day after I made this decision, I woke up at 4 a.m. I like to say Spirit energy kicked my butt out of bed and got me writing at my desk. Me, write? What will I say? "This is not a big deal that I am going grey. Many have gone grey before me. Books have been written. Facebook and Instagram groups have been formed. I'm too late. I should have written my book when I was thirty-five, you chicken shit."

Negative self-talk was filling my head and I needed to stop. How would I be able to write a book if I let my negative thoughts run my life? You know those self-sabotaging thoughts that keep us from living our best lives. You probably have them running through your head right now and you don't even notice. "I could never write." "I'm not smart enough." "I'm too fat." "I'm too lazy." "I'm stupid." "I'm not pretty enough." "I'm not skinny enough." "No one loves me." "I never have enough money." "I hate my job." "My house is too small." You get my point! I want you to catch yourself with these negative thoughts and write them down. I want you to figure out where these thoughts come from. Then reword those thoughts and create a new story and meaning around them. Why is this an important exercise? Because these thoughts are ruling your life at a subconscious level. They are probably keeping you stuck at the same job, with the same income, and the same okay life. These thoughts are holding you back from greatness. Would you not want to dig deeper and change it? I know I wanted a different life. Average to me was boring. I wanted an above-average life, and I was the only person standing in the way of achieving that goal. Following is an exercise I did to help change my negative thinking. You can do it for yourself as well:

1. What is a negative thought that keeps showing up for you?

   My answer: I can't write.

2. Why do you think this negative thought keeps coming up?

   My answer: Fear that I'm not good enough. Fear of telling the world my story and being judged. Fear of failure.

3. What "story" have you connected this negative thought too?

   My answer: English was my worst subject. I hated reading. I hated writing even more. My teacher told me I was a terrible writer, so I believed her. I was hiding my voice from the world because it felt safe.

4. Are you willing to give up the story and create a new one?

   My answer: Yes. I am scared, but my desire is now bigger than my fear.

6. What would your new story sound like?

   My answer: I am a writer. I have my own style. I am unique. I have a voice. I am good enough. I believe I can make a difference.

I will share more of my stories with you later in this chapter so you will understand how I had to change my script to get to the place where I could go grey and write this book.

Let's go back to October 2018. Hours after I started writing, I was inspired to set up a Facebook support group, and I called it the "Gorgeous Grey Movement." I wanted to start a movement of women who had been thinking about going grey but were scared like me, as well as women who had gone before me and were brave enough to share their stories and inspire us. I designed the logo and opened up the Facebook group on a Saturday morning. It was a fast process. I felt I was divinely guided. I was going with the flow. It was easy. By the end of the weekend, one hundred women had joined. This was the sign I needed to keep going. I was committed and I wanted to make a difference. Some women who joined were already grey and had gone before us. I call them my mentors. My Grey-Hair Heroes. The women who had to dig into their core and conquer their fears and say *yes*. A lot of them did this before the time that grey was a trend—before social media and all the "grey" hype. A big shout out to all the Grey-Hair Heroes who have gone before me! You are the shoulder I lean on in this transition. You are the brave souls who have shown your vulnerability to the world. You are rebels.

When I saw the trailer for the film *Grey Is the New Blonde*, I was so excited that a documentary was coming out to showcase this movement of women embracing grey. In the trailer I heard the producer say, "When you go out to the world and see a woman sporting at least four inches of grey, you know she is a *bad ass*." I loved that awakening. It carries me through the more challenging days when I feel I look like a skunk. I replace my stinking thinking with, "*I am a bad ass.*" I am writing this four months into my transition. I have good-hair days and bad-hair days. When I see pictures come up on Facebook as a reminder of what happened one year ago, and see pictures of the old Nicole, fear comes up. Fear of not looking good and put together. Fear of looking older than my age. I often have to remind myself why I started this new journey. My Gorgeous Grey Movement support group helps me through these fears. I have no problem asking for help and encouragement on the tough days. Who do you turn to for support and encouragement? Whatever your struggles are in life, do you have people you can lean on and be vulnerable with? I have learned that there are so many support groups to help you through your darkest days. You don't have to be alone in your struggles. Learn to ask for help. There are good people waiting to hear your story who genuinely want to help.

Ask yourself why you want to go grey. What are your deepest fears that are holding you back? Where does that fear come from? Every time a new member joins the Gorgeous Grey Movement, they answer this question: "What is your biggest fear of going grey? The top responses are (1) looking older than I am, (2) that grey won't look good on me, and (3) my family won't support me.

You see, most women and probably most men have the same fears, all based on how they will look. It's being human. It's being human with fears. Not everyone has these fears; some women answer, "Bring it on. I am ready!" We are all motivated and inspired by different experiences.

If we don't overcome our fear of eventually going grey, then where else in our lives could we be hiding from fear? You see, it's not just about going grey that we fear, it shows up in other areas of our lives too. If I hadn't crushed other fears in my life, I don't think I could have gone grey. Going grey was so scary, and I had so much meaning attached to it. If I hadn't done the work on myself before this journey, I believe I would still be dyeing my hair black every three weeks. Here are a few examples of my fears and limiting beliefs that I had to overcome. Can you relate to any of them?

- Fear of a new relationship. "Love hurts! Maybe I will never find love again."
- Fear of moving. "Having to say goodbye hurts! It's hard finding new friends."
- Fear of speaking in front of people. "People will judge me. I will embarrass myself."
- Fear of having a network-marketing business. "What will people think? Does it really work?"

I could go on and on about fears because I think we all have them. Some have a longer list than others. I have been doing personal development since I was a teenager, thanks to Tony Robbins cassette tapes that my mom forced me to listen to on long road trips to visit family.

Once I was clear on my *why* for going grey, it got easier to have conversations with people about my decision. The feedback I was getting from others was mostly positive and supportive. The biggest response I got from women was, "You're brave," or "Wow, I could never do that." I giggle inside because I know what they mean. That would probably have been my response a year ago, before my journey began.

If I can share in my vulnerability around my fears, maybe it will help others overcome theirs as well. We live in a society where youth is rewarded and marketed everywhere. We are fighting a deeply embedded societal behaviour of anti-aging. No wonder fear enters the equation of our decision to go grey. The negative self-doubt conversation begins: "Will I fit in?" "Will I look pretty enough?" "Will I be accepted?"

"Will I look older?" "Will I feel good about myself?" "Will my partner like it?" These are all our deepest fears showing up in one decision. Holy crap! Who would have thought! Just when you think you've done enough personal-development work to deal with all your past demons—nope, they show up again to remind you the work must continue.

As my transition to grey unfolded, I actually started to get more and more excited about the journey. I wasn't giving as much attention to the fear anymore, but more to the possibilities. "What if I actually looked hot and sexy?" "What if my health improved?" "What if I inspired a bigger movement?" "What if I really liked who I am with my new sparkle?" "What if my partner accepted all of me?" "What if my kids finally embraced the change?" "What if I gained more grey-haired friends?" "What if …?" You can see how this change in thoughts can really start to *win* the battle.

Friends began to say to me, "OMG, Nicole, are you actually going to go grey? Are you sure you want to do this? Why don't you wait, you look so sexy and youthful with your long dark hair? If you don't like it you can just change it back." Most of my friends were supportive, whereas others questioned how long I would last. Well, let's go back thirteen years to when this idea arose.

I was thirty-five years old, in the shower washing another home-dye kit off my head, watching it drip down onto my breasts, over my belly, and down my legs. I was thinking, "Really, Nicole, this must not be good for you. How many chemicals are you putting into your body and your brain each month because you want to look younger? You have been dyeing your hair for over five years already—when do you think you will stop?"

My mom dyed her hair for a good twenty-plus years before she said no more and went fully grey at age fifty-three. I told myself, "I'm too young to go grey—OMG! Your husband [at the time] still gets asked for ID at the liquor store, and you're thinking about going grey. Are you out of your mind? People will think you are his mother. Is that what you want? *No.* He will leave you and you will never be able to find a man at thirty-five with grey hair, so get over yourself and dye your hair already."

I started to get that taste on my tongue right away—that toxic tongue taste as if my body were screaming at me to stop the toxic load *for real* this time. I'm a nutritionist; I know better. It's all about keeping the toxic load low and supporting liver health. I justified it with, "It's only once a month, and I buy as natural as I can. That has to count for something, right?" I came up with a book idea in the shower. I wrote it down in my journal and that was it. I was going to write a book on going grey in my thirties. I told myself, "This could be *big*! Imagine coming out of the closet at thirty-five and telling the world 'I am grey!' Is the world ready for a grey thirty-year-old?" This moment in the shower was a wake-up call for me, but I was not ready to fully listen to my body or answer that call until years later when I had a health scare.

There was no social media at that time, and it was hard to find mentors. I remember I was at the cottage and went to the gym. I dropped the girls off at daycare and ran into a lady in the change room who was fully grey (I was thirty-five), and she looked great. I was brave enough to ask her—after I complimented her on how awesome she looked with her grey hair, "How old are you?"

"Really, Nicole?" I said to myself, "You asked her how old she was? How dare you? Who cares how old she is? Does it really matter?" I guess to me, I was so worried about how going grey aged us that I was fixated on knowing her age. She told me she was forty. Wow, I was inspired! Maybe I could do this at age thirty-five. Why did I have so much fear? Fear of looking old, fear of people judging me, fear of people thinking I was a grandma to my kids, fear of not getting noticed again. OMG, I had so many fears. And those fears kept me from dyeing my hair over and over and over again.

I did the calculations. If, at age thirty, when I started going grey, I began dyeing my hair approximately once a month for seventeen years, that would equal 204 dye jobs. Lots of those dye jobs would be done in-home because they're much less expensive, but some would be done in a salon. Holy moly, can you spend a fortune in a hair salon! I know that over the last four years I had to go approximately every three weeks to a salon to cover up. That means that seventeen visits a year at $120 per visit over four years would cost $8,160, and that was on the less expensive side. I remember being charged over $200 at a higher-end salon.

How was I going to hide that expense from my hubby (now ex)? That was a week's worth of groceries. Have you ever had to hide your hair bill from your partner because you knew it was way out of your budget? My sister just recently told me she would get a bill for $300 from a senior stylist. My point is that you could certainly save a lot of money embracing grey and save it for something else, such as a dream vacation or a down payment on a cottage. I guess it really does come down to our value system and how we spend to match our values. No judgment, but looking back, a dream vacation with family sounded good to me. Memories that last forever—sign me up for that! I dare you to do a rough estimate of how much money you have spent dyeing your hair over the years. Would you spend it differently? If I had to do it all over again, I would have let the grey come in and own that sparkle. I would have saved money and time and reduced my toxic load. The amount of money I spent dyeing my hair was a wake-up call for sure!

So why did it take me so long to come out of the closet and declare, "I am going grey"? Fear, fear, fear. It's so ironic to me that I can feel the fear and do it anyway on so many levels in my life, but going grey paralyzed me. I ask myself, "What is the deal, Nicole? How have you conquered so much fear in your life, Nicole?"

Good and bad things happen to all of us. After experiencing an emotional event, we create a story about it that has the potential to become part of our operating system as we move through life. So, depending on the story we create (good or bad), it can really have a huge impact on how our lives turn out. I learned this concept back in my early thirties, when I took an amazing personal-development program called the Landmark Forum. It transformed me in so many ways. It was another wake-up call to personal growth. It helped me to understand my pain stories—stories that I made up as a child and teenager—and how they were running my life. My inner child/teen was truly running the show in my adult life. Kind of sounds crazy, right? But it was true. Guess what I had to do? I wrote down all the pain stories that I remembered and reflected on the ones that I created around those events, asking myself if this was the story that was running my life. Wow! Talk about peeling the layers off the onion—I had no idea that there were so many darn stories. This is a great exercise for anyone to do. I dare you to dig deep and find out where your stories originated from. You might be as surprised as I was to discover that an eight-year-old girl was running my show.

Following is another exercise that I did; this one regarding a childhood experience that I remember as being painful. This example shows how I had to work through this pain story. I encourage you to do this exercise by coming up with at least three stories of your own—since most of us have more than one—of pain or embarrassment.

What is your pain story?
A close family member tried to commit suicide when I was in grade 3. It was the most traumatic experience of my childhood.

What story did you create around that event that is now part of your operating system?
This event was my fault. If I had been better behaved. If I'd stopped fighting with my sister. If I had helped out more, this would not have happened. I blamed myself (that little eight-year-old girl). So the story that became part of my operating system was, "I am not good enough. Keep the peace. Don't cause conflict and do everything you are told to do." This was the story I believed and why I gave up my voice in the world because of the fear that I would hurt someone.

What new story could replace the old story?
I told myself it wasn't my fault. I was eight years old. This family member was an adult and totally responsible for their actions. I was a child of divine energy, and I was given a voice to speak the truth, my truth. The world needs to hear from me. I am safe. I am good enough.

With this personal example you can see how easily a story can be created in a young person's mind, and how it can contribute very easily to your new operating system in the future. This story impacted me on so many levels because I avoided conflict with everyone. I didn't have a voice. I gave my power away and just backed down on everything. I let people, especially men, walk all over me. I didn't know how to speak my truth.

My sister, Tracy, was a firecracker who found her voice and told everyone her truth and then some. To say I was jealous of her was an understatement. How could she be so bold, so brave, to just say what was on her mind? She obviously never created a story around that emotional event like I did. It's fascinating to me how powerful this story was for me but not for her.

I mentioned not speaking my truth. What body part is impacted by not speaking our truth? The throat. Later in life, I would learn about the chakras. What is the chakra system? The seven chakras are the energy centres in our bodies that energy flows through. The word *chakra* is derived from the Sanskrit word meaning "wheel." A chakra is like a whirling, vortex-like powerhouse of energy. Within our bodies, we have seven major energy centres and many more minor ones. In Sanskrit, the word *Vishuddha* (meaning "purification") is used for the fifth chakra—the throat chakra. This chakra is the centre of communication as it is located between the third and fifth vertebrae in the neck and opens towards the throat. Centrally, it lies at the base of the neck. Chakras can become blocked through an emotional upset, such as conflict, loss, or accident. Fear, anxiety, and stress are common causes of chakra malfunction. These blocks disrupt harmony in our bodies, eventually becoming the cause of disease, as well as emotional and mental disorders. *You Can Heal Your Life* by Louise Hay is a great book to learn more about the mind-body connection.

Where do you think a lot of my problems happened in my body? You guessed it, my mouth. I had constant throat infections and a buildup of mucus that caused me to clear my throat often. Mucus is not a cool thing to have as a young girl as it made me have to spit often, which was very embarrassing. One early morning after breastfeeding Sydney, I broke my two front teeth when I passed out while sitting on the toilet. Smash! Down I went, face first on the tile. I bit right through my lip and blood was everywhere. Because I had the flu bug, my period, and I had just finished breastfeeding, I had nothing left in my body to nourish me and down I went. I believe this event was a scream for help, but I didn't know how to ask for help because I had no voice. I learned to suck it up. I had to do everything myself. I had to show the world how tough I was. Does this sound familiar to anyone?

Luckily, my mom was staying with us at the time, and she realized how much help I needed with two young children and my family spread out across the country. My mom made a joke, "You know you could have just asked for help instead of breaking your teeth." Like those Tony Robbins personal-development tapes, mom came through again, introducing me to Louise Hay's book. Mom was really into her teachings and understood the connection between how blocked chakras can impact the body.

Years later, I developed a massive infection in a bottom back tooth that caused a lot of discomfort and many trips to the dentist. We tried to save the tooth, but it was too infected and had to be extracted. Again, looking back at that time in my life, there was a lot that had been left unsaid in my marriage. Sucking it up was better than dealing with the conflict was my mantra. How many of us have learned to suck it up and hold back the truth? Who taught us this? Our parents? Our society? Our stories we created to protect ourselves? I paid the price for holding back as it caused a lot of emotional pain that I could have avoided if I had understood the story that was controlling my life. Some of you may not believe that connection—I get it. It took me a long time to get my head wrapped around this theory, but over the years, as I took notice, it became more and more clear that there seemed to be a huge connection between the mind and body. Where in your body is there emotional pain? What story could you be holding on to that is causing your physical pain?

> *"The greater part of human pain is unnecessary. It is self-created as long as the unobserved mind runs your life."*
> —ECKHART TOLLE

Who is running the show? Can you get tuned in to the stories that are holding you back? My new-found awareness of how my stories ruled me allowed me to be more kind to and more compassionate with myself and others. My relationships improved and my positive attitude started to shine brighter. Here are some of the tools I use to stay on top of my stories and help crush my fears:

Meditation/Prayer

A morning ritual of meditation keeps me grounded and connected to divine energy. I light a candle with an essential oil (bergamot is my favourite) and spend just a few minutes in gratitude and stillness. I fill my heart up with love and visualize a white light coming in from my crown and moving through me. I ask for guidance and connection. This calmness allows me to start my day with a grateful heart full of love. How do you start your day? Do you give yourself some quiet time to gather your thoughts and visualize a day full of possibilities? Try starting with just a few minutes a day, even before you jump out of bed. Ask yourself, "What am I grateful for? How can I be of service to others? How can I show myself self-love today?" Starting your day with the right positive mindset can help you control your fears that start to take over before you even get out of bed.

Yoga/Breath Practice

Whenever something comes up as a trigger, I practise taking three deep breaths before I react. It grounds me and gives me enough time to decide my next move without the potential of overreacting. I am not perfect, but this tool has helped save me from many embarrassing child-like behaviours that want to come out kicking and screaming. Researchers have found that meditating and breathing techniques result in an improved immune system and can literally change your brain's wiring. "Breath-focused meditation and yogic breathing practices have numerous known cognitive benefits, including increased ability to focus, decreased mind wandering, improved arousal levels, more positive emotions, decreased emotional reactivity, along with many others."[1] Who would have thought that breath could be so important to our mental health? How are you breathing right now? Do you need to take three deep breaths and ground yourself?

Gratitude

There are many ways you can show gratitude in a day. Prayer at night. Grace at dinner. Thanking someone for their help or gifts. I have a few rituals of gratitude with my family. At dinnertime when we are all together (very rare these days), we share one thing we are grateful for about the day. I also have a journal and write down at least three things that I am grateful for about the day, or at least communicate that with my partner before we fall asleep. Studies have shown that the mere act of thanking someone can be good for your health. For example, a study published in *Journal of Happiness Studies* found that those who wrote letters of gratitude over a three-week period were happier, had greater life satisfaction, and had less incidence of depressive symptoms.[2] How many times a day do you show gratitude to others? Whom could you send a note to right now to tell them how grateful you are for having them in your life? After you have sent the note, notice how you feel. I know when I get a special note of gratitude from someone it makes me smile and warms my heart.

Affirmations

I have several affirmation cards scattered around my house. My favourite cards are from a friend of mine, Lorna Lahav, called *I Am* cards (see the resources section on page 235). They are cards that I grab each day to remind me of my greatness. As we go about our day and negativity shows up, it's easy to forget the positive *you*. Affirmation cards are a great tool to stay in the zone of your "greatness." Here is a card that I pulled out for you today:

I am committed.

Today I will set one important goal and stick to it. I will do this in order to move forward and be in accordance with my own standards. Focusing on the past will not build the future. I will clear my mind. Start with a clean state and cut a blazing path.

I will succeed.

If you don't have a deck of affirmation cards, it may be time to invest in one. Just another tool to keep you in the positive zone.

Feel My Fear and Do It Anyway

This was a coaching moment by my mentor, Dr. Mitra Ray, years ago when I was learning to build my online wellness franchise. She was always asking me to be teachable. I resisted big time. I wanted to do it my way because it felt safe and familiar, but guess what—it was not growing my business. I remember that she taught us a new way to close a sale. She called it the "ABC Close Technique." It terrified me. I still remember practising it for the first time in a basement of a friend's house. She had ten women over, and I was presenting a talk on wellness. It was time to close. My heart started racing, my face turned bright red, and I felt as if I wanted to puke. All I could hear was Mitra's voice telling me to be teachable if I wanted to grow. I barely got through the close, but I did it. I am sure it was horrible, and I made everyone just as uncomfortable as I was. I did tell them I was new at this, so please give me some grace. Well, we did get one order out of the presentation, so I guess it wasn't a total flop. What I learned from that experience, however, was that it empowered me to want to practise so I could get better and better. Now I can't imagine not using the ABC Close. It feels good and authentic. I can now teach others how to be confident at closing the sale with grace and ease. Remember, it was a huge fear, but with enough practise it became easy. I have so many examples of stories of overcoming my fears, and I'm sure you do too.

Write down five stories in your life where you overcame fear and it turned out okay, or even better than okay. What did you learn from that experience?

You see, we need to remember those stories of overcoming fear so it can to lead us to our next chapters in life. I am grateful for all the "fear stories" I had to crush, because without them I wouldn't be here writing this book. Is it your time to crush your fear around going grey and just do it, like I did?

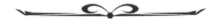

"Our deepest fear is not that we are inadequate. Our deepest fear is that we are powerful beyond measure. It is our light, not our darkness that most frightens us. We ask ourselves, who am I to be brilliant, gorgeous, talented, and fabulous? Actually, who are you not to be? You are a child of God. Your playing small does not serve the world. There is nothing enlightened about shrinking so that other people won't feel insecure around you. We are all meant to shine, as children do. We were born to make manifest the glory of God that is within us. It's not just in some of us; it's in everyone. And as we let our own light

shine, we unconsciously give other people permission to do the same. As we are liberated from our own fear, our presence automatically liberates others."[3]

—MARIANNE WILLIAMSON

CHAPTER SIX

Healthy Hair at Any Age

"I am not beautiful like you. I am beautiful like me."

—Author unknown

Who wants healthy hair? Me please! Ask any women about what is important to them in beauty care, and hair health usually lands on top of the list. Our hair seems to define us in so many ways. So much so that we can even label a person just by a glance at their hair. What attachment do you have to your hair? How do you let it define who you are? When I had kids, I kept my hair really short for ease. Wash and go! My boyfriend jokes when he sees old pictures and calls it my "soccer-mom hair." Can anyone relate to that? When I got divorced, I decided I was going to grow it out long. I wanted to feel sexy again, and somehow I attached long hair with that image of sexy. Did I feel different about myself with long hair? Yes. I felt sexy and youthful with longer hair. I also think I felt this way because I was doing a ton of self-care and spiritual work to change my mindset. I used to go weekly to get my hair professionally straightened, and every three weeks to cover my grey. Nothing feels better than a polished mane of hair. My hair glowed and it grew fast. It was healthy. I got so many compliments about how healthy my hair looked. I used organic products to wash my hair, washed it only once a week, and let it dry naturally. Long hair was easy to take care of, except for the root touch-ups. In this chapter I want to share with you what it takes to have healthy hair, the transition strategy I chose to go grey, and some tips from some of my hairstylists.

As a nutritionist for fourteen years, my focus has been all about supporting clients' overall health from the inside out, but I never focused on hair health specifically. Healthy hair, skin, and nails eventually showed up for my clients once we cleaned up their diet, added tons of plants, detoxed them, and added the right supplements to support their body's needs. This process doesn't happen overnight. Dr. Michael Colgan writes in *Optimum Sports Nutrition*: "Unlike drugs, nutrients do not have rapid effects. No quick fix. The business of nutrition is to build a better body. That has to wait on nature to turn over body cells. A blood cell lasts 60-120 days. In 3-4 months, your whole blood supply is completely replaced. In 6 months almost all of the proteins in your body die and are replaced, even the DNA in your genes. In a year, all of your bones and even the enamel on your teeth is replaced, constructed entirely out of the nutrients you eat. Think of it this way: if you take a neglected houseplant and start feeding and watering it, the leaves may perk up a bit from the improved nutrition. But you have to wait for the old leaves to die off and new leaves to grow before you get a really healthy plant. It is the same with the human body. When you start feeding it better, you have to wait on your body to grow new improved cells."[1]

My point here is that there is no easy quick fix for healthy hair. It takes time and effort. You can temporarily put on the putty and the oils to make it look healthy like I had to do. Why the putty? Because it hides all the breakage—those small pieces that stick up all over the place. I never had to use hair putty until I got breakage from overbleaching. It was a great tool to tame my hair. Natural Oils such as coconut oil, neem oil and argan oil have helped put some life back into my dry brittle hair. Purple shampoo has also helped take some of the green out of my hair after a dip in a chlorinated pool. Silly me. What was I thinking? Chlorine and bleach don't work well together, ladies, so watch your hair when you go swimming. If you are on well water there are a lot of metals that can very quickly change your bleached hair to unwanted colours, so that is where blue or purple shampoos will save you from looking like a green-haired monster. My new natural hair coming in looks so healthy and gives me hope that in less than a year I will be able to cut the remaining bleached and coloured pieces out and be free of the dye forever.

Have you ever considered that the health of your hair and nails is a good indicator of your general wellbeing? Diet plays the biggest factor in achieving healthy hair. Are you happy with your hair health? If not, we need to take a closer look at your diet and your stress levels. Since our hair is composed largely of keratin protein, good-quality proteins such as beans with whole grains, eggs, seeds, collagen, and fish play a key role in achieving healthy hair. Let's take a look deep into the hair follicle. "A hair follicle anchors each hair into the skin. In the hair bulb, living cells divide and grow to build the hair shaft. Blood vessels nourish the cells in the hair bulb, and deliver *hormones* [emphasis mine] that modify hair growth and structure at different times of life."[2] We need to treat our hair just as we would our skin. We need to nourish it, hydrate it, and protect it. Healthy hair starts from within. Did you know that our skin is our largest organ? That what we put on our skin we absorb? You want to choose wisely. That is why I am such an advocate for clean organic products in the kitchen as well as the products we use in the bathroom for our bodies. Often women don't pay attention to the level of toxins that are lurking in the bathroom. Turn your hair products around and read the label to see what they are full of. The products you use on your body are just as important as those you put in your body. Fewer toxins equals a healthier functioning body, and the good news is that we can control what we eat and what we put on our bodies.

I had a few clients whose hair was falling out, and I put them on a four-month whole-food program with supplements, and within sixteen weeks their bald spots started to fill in and their hair stopped falling out. One client's grey hair reversed itself by changing her diet—obviously, there were nutritional deficiencies that we were able to fill in with some extra supplements and clean eating. How cool is that? Having healthy hair is usually a result of a healthy diet, they go hand in hand. However, there is a genetic factor that impacts earlier greying that plays a role as well. If your parents' or grandparents' hair turned grey at an early age, yours probably will too. Hair follicles contain pigment cells that produce melanin, which gives your hair its colour. Grey hair occurs, in part, when the body starts producing less melanin. When and how much melanin the body produces is determined by genetics. The good news is that scientists have pinpointed exactly which gene may be responsible for this colour change. When your body stops producing melanin, hair starts turning white, silver, or grey.

"As hair greys something happens that causes this gene to produce even lower levels of melanin. Now we can ask more specific functional questions."[3] And asking the right questions will bring them a step closer to identifying therapies that delay the greying of hair. A company that I partnered with in Toronto, The DNA Company, is on the cutting edge of DNA and custom-made supplements to support better health. This would be a great option for people with early grey or balding to consider as a preventive strategy. I wonder if I had started this DNA journey twenty years ago I could have delayed my grey sparkle until my eighties—hmm. I have been on their custom-made supplements for about a year to help me address my estrogen dominance, and I love how I feel. Getting my DNA analysis done and having a consultation with them was so empowering. I believe this will be the future of medicine. Still, genetics isn't necessarily destiny. Dr. Adhikari figures that the IRF4 gene variant accounts for about 30% of grey hair, with environmental factors—including, perhaps, stress—accounting for the rest.[4] Whether or not you decide to invest in a DNA analysis like I did, the best place to start would be to take a look at your lifestyle and focus on adopting a whole-food diet to impact your overall health, and the bonus will be healthier hair.

What to Consider When Looking at Your Diet to Improve Your Hair Health

1. *Vitamins, Minerals, and Antioxidants*

Get your blood work done to confirm any deficiencies. Your medical doctor can order the basic testing to start your investigation. I prefer to use my naturopath doctor for advanced blood testing and live blood analysis.

Learn whether you are deficient in key vitamins and minerals such as zinc and iron. Both are essential for hair growth. Zinc is responsible for shiny hair, and when your body is depleted in this mineral, your strands can look dull and even grey. Iron deficiency is linked to hair loss in men and in women, as well as iron-deficiency anemia. Iron helps carry oxygen to hair follicles, and when there isn't enough, hair loss occurs. When my daughter was iron depleted (because of a parasite), her hair was falling out by the handful and it stopped growing. As soon as we put her on a parasite cleanse and got her iron count up through supplementation and cleaning up her diet, we started to see her hair health come around and she began to feel much better.

The good news is that these essential nutrients are fairly easy to get from your diet since they are found in so many delicious foods: nuts, seeds, millet, quinoa, beans, lentils, green leafy vegetables, fruits, eggs, and animal proteins. If you're eating a varied, rainbow-colored, heavily plant-based whole-food diet, you're already getting lots of these nutrients every day. One of my favourite tools that I recommend for clients and give to my family is a plant-based food concentrate in a capsule called Juice Plus+ that helps bridge any daily gap in fruits, vegetables, and berries. Most of my clients have great intentions to hit 10+ servings a day of fruits and vegetables, but in reality most of them don't. The USDA Food Guide and the Canada Food Guide recommend filling half your plate with fruits and vegetables as part of a balanced diet. That would be approximately seven to 10+ servings a day. Researchers estimated that approximately 7.8 million premature deaths worldwide may be prevented every year if people eat 10 portions of fruits and vegetables a day.[5] In 2004, Canadians reported having about 5.2 servings of fruit and vegetables a day, but by 2015, they were eating just 4.6 servings daily.[6] In 2017 in the US, only 1 out of 10 adults are meeting the daily recommendation.[7] These stats are alarming and show us how big the gap really is. How many plants a day are you eating? How about your children? Do you need to fill in your gap by taking the simple step of adding more color to each plate for the health of it? Just by increasing your intake of plants you will not only reduce your risk of disease but the results will also start to show up in your hair, skin, and nails.

2. *Protein*

Our hair follicles are made up mostly of protein, and that means getting enough of it will help keep your hair healthy and strong. Good sources of protein are essential for healthy hair and skin. Protein-deficient diets are linked to hair loss and thinning.

I have personal experience with hair loss due to lack of nutrition, including protein, when I was in high school. When I moved to another city in my final year, I met a new friend who had an eating disorder from trying to stay thin. I was also desperate to keep my weight low and felt so much peer pressure to be thin, so I joined her. Very quickly my health started going downhill. My hair began to fall out by the handful, I was tired all the time, and I was as pale as a ghost. My poor body was starving for nutrition, and it was starting to show up in my appearance. My mom caught me one day in the bathroom after months of throwing up after all my meals. She freaked out and taught me about the long-term dangers of this behaviour to my health. When she told me that all my hair could fall out and I could ruin my teeth, I stopped immediately. She woke me up. I had to rebuild a new relationship to food—and build up my health again. Over time

I healed from the eating disorder and got my health back. Today I am thirty pounds heavier than I was in high school before and after my eating disorder, and I'm okay with that. I have learned to love my body and not define myself by the weight scale. I feel healthy and energized. That is more important to me than the number on the scale. How attached are you to the scale? Does it hold you prisoner? Is it time to start focusing on health rather than a number?

What proteins can you add to your diet? Good, clean sources could include spirulina, a blue-green algae that contains about 60% protein and can be added to a morning smoothie; whole grains, nuts, seeds, wild-caught fish, plant-based protein powders, free-run poultry, eggs, pastured meat, a collagen supplement, and bone broth. Everyone in my family starts their day with a shake full of plant proteins, fruits, and vegetables. Here are two of our favourite whole-food protein-shake recipes:

Chocolate Monkey

1 frozen banana

1 tablespoon (15 mL) nut butter (almond, cashew, or peanut)

1 tablespoon (15 mL) seeds (hemp, chia, or flax)

1 scoop plant-based protein powder (chocolate flavour; Juice Plus+ Complete is my favourite)

1 to 2 cups (250–500 mL) plant milk (almond, hemp, oat, or rice), depending on how thick you like your shake; start with 1 cup (250 mL), and then you can always add more

1 handful greens (organic kale or spinach)

Optional:

Serious chocolate lovers can add 1 tablespoon (15 mL) of Organic Cacao Nibs (or powder), a superfood made by Organic traditions.

Combine all the ingredients in a food processor and blend for 30 seconds. Enjoy.

Vanilla Beach

1 cup (250 mL) frozen mixed tropical fruits (mango, pineapple, and banana)

1 tablespoon (15 mL) seeds (hemp, chia, or flax)

1 scoop plant-based protein powder (vanilla flavour Juice Plus+ is my favourite)

1 handful greens (organic kale or spinach)

1 to 2 cups (250–500 mL) plant milk (almond, hemp, oat, or rice), depending on how thick you like your shake; start with 1 cup (250 mL), and then you can always add more

Optional:

1 teaspoon (5 mL) turmeric, a superfood

Combine all the ingredients in a food processor and blend for 30 seconds. Enjoy.

3. *Healthy Fats*

Thank goodness the low-fat craze is over, and new evidence has built up over the years that we need healthy fats to thrive, especially if you want to have healthy hair and skin. Since our bodies don't produce the essential fatty acids (EFAs), omega-3 and omega-6 fatty acids, which are critical for overall health, we need to get them every day from our diets. Why are EFAs so important? They support many functions in our bodies, such as increasing the absorption of vitamins and minerals; nourishing the skin, hair, and nails; promoting proper nerve function; helping to produce hormones; and ensuring normal growth and development.[8,9]

We can find these fats in avocados, nuts, seeds, and coconut oil. Essential fatty acids have the ability to turn dry, brittle hair into a stronger and lush head of hair by nourishing from the roots to strengthen our hair as it grows. I have never been a great fan of taking fatty acid supplements because they have to be refrigerated, and they can go rancid or taste fishy, and I found they made me burp. To be honest, I thought that I was getting enough EFAs from my diet, and I didn't need to supplement. However, last year I experimented by adding a plant-based EFA supplement to my daily diet. This product was shelf-stable, so I could take it with me wherever I went. I soon began to notice a huge change in my hair health, such as thicker hair that grew faster, with the bonus that my brain and joint health improved as well. Even my teenage girls noticed how much faster their hair grew. So it seemed that we weren't getting enough EFAs in our diet and supplementation was necessary. This shocked me because we had fish, which are rich in EFAs, at least twice a week. We also ate tons of nuts and seeds, and avocados almost daily.

"According to CHMS [Canadian Health Measures Survey] results, 2.6% of Canadians aged 20 to 79 met the Omega-3 Index level associated with low risk of CHD [coronary heart disease], and 43% were in the high-risk category."[10] In addition, a study in 2014 showed that "U.S. adults are not meeting recommended levels for fish and omega-3 fatty acid intake."[11] Looking at the statistics of Canada and the United States, we can see that there is a huge fatty-acid deficiency that needs to be filled. In my professional opinion, I would recommend a fatty-acid supplement for my clients on top of a whole-food diet.

Factors that Impact Hair Health and Going Grey Early

Nutritional Deficiencies

Any deficiencies of vitamin B-6, B-12, biotin, vitamin D, or vitamin E can contribute to premature greying. A 2015 report in the journal *Development* notes various deficiency studies on vitamin D3, vitamin B12, and copper and their connection to greying hair. It finds that nutritional deficiencies affect pigmentation, suggesting that colour can return with vitamin supplementation.[12]

Smoking

Early greying or not smoking? You choose. A study from 2013 reported in the *Italian Dermatology Online* Journal showed that smokers are 2½ times more likely to start greying before age thirty as non-smokers.[13] And a 2015 study in the *Journal of the American Academy of Dermatology* also demonstrated that smoking is linked to premature white hair in young men.[14]

Stress Level

Science has mixed reviews about whether or not stress is directly linked to grey hair. If it impacts your hair colour or not, I know for sure that high stress has sent me into adrenal burnout and depression. Not a fun place to be. One study from New York University, reported in *Nature Medicine, finds that the cells responsible for hair colour can be depleted when the body is under stress.*[15] When you're constantly stressed or struggling with an anxiety disorder, you're more likely to find grey hairs before your more relaxed peers do. Furthermore, there is plenty of anecdotal evidence to suggest that stress is indeed related to the greying process.

According to an article in *Scientific American,* a traumatic event can affect your whole body—even damaging your hair follicles.[16] Basically, an incredibly stressful event can generate a swarm of free radicals in your hair follicles that travel along the hair shaft, destroying its pigment in a manner that appears similar to a bleaching effect.

Learning to manage your stress will benefit your entire body in the long run. Some of the stress reduction techniques I have used over the years have been mediation, walking in nature, writing, and talking to a friend.

Medical Conditions

Occasionally, an underlying medical condition could be to blame for early greying. Some autoimmune and genetic conditions have been linked to premature greying. As well, if you have diabetes, pernicious anemia, or thyroid problems, these illnesses are known for directly attacking your hair follicles.[17] Check with your healthcare professional to make sure you don't have an underlying medical condition.

Too Much Sun

If you want shiny, soft, and healthy hair, keeping it protected from the sun is essential. Just like SPF for skin, we need to consider a protection formula to protect our hair from the sun. I had never thought that I needed sunscreen for my hair, but now it sure makes sense. UV rays affect your hair follicles. In short, it has a bleaching effect on your hair that's incredibly damaging, leaving your follicles brittle and prone to breakage, resulting in the replacement of your healthy strands with grey ones. If you have grey hair like me and you love the sun, you are at risk of getting sun damage. Make sure you not only spray your hair with protection but also wear a hat. Look for sun-protection products that contain natural ingredients, such as coconut oil or shea butter and state that they protect from UV damage. A quick spray on your hair in the morning can be a great step to protecting your beautiful mane.

Overstyling

What tools do you use to style your hair? Could they be contributing to your sizzled hair? Blow-dryers and hot styling tools such as flat irons and curlers can contribute to damaged hair. Heat that is too hot can literally form bubbles on the hair shaft, making the hair coarse and promoting breakage. One of my grey-hair mentors on YouTube showed us how she burned her grey hair using a flat iron. Her hair went from a beautiful grey sparkle to a bunch of yellow patches all over her head, just because the flat iron was too hot. Turn down the heat, ladies! You will also want to use a heat protection spray on your hair before you use a hot styling tool. Look for tools with ionic or ceramic technology that dry the hair using much less heat than traditional tools. There's no way around it: Using bleach to lift hair colour will weaken hair bonds, leading to drier texture and damage. My hairstylist uses Olaplex—a favourite treatment that's worked into the colouring process to reconnect broken disulfide sulfur bonds for a healthier result (see the resources section on page 235).

Hormones

We women love to blame everything on our hormones. I am as guilty as anyone else. Cramps – hormones. Tender breasts – hormones. Mood swings – hormones. Muffin top – hormones. Wrinkles – hormones. Tired – hormones. Hair loss – hormones, and the list goes on and on. There is a lot of truth to the notion that our health issues, including our hair health, can be impacted by our hormones. I reached out to one of my mentors, Jenn Pike, who specializes in women's hormones, to shed some light on the impact hormones have on our hair health. Following is her professional advice.

We all know that our hormones affect many processes in the body from our menstrual cycle and menopause to our weight, mood, and energy, but did you know that your hormonal health also impacts your hair health?

If you're suffering from lowered estrogen, this can cause dry hair and increased hair loss, while higher estrogen can cause oily, greasy hair. If you're suffering from elevated androgens (testosterone and DHEA), you are more likely to suffer from rapidly thinning hair on your head but excess hair growth on your chin, face, chest, and navel. From your years in puberty through your high fertility years, pregnancy, postpartum, perimenopause, menopause, and beyond, your hair as a woman goes through many hormonally induced changes. What are some of the key changes you may notice?

- Thinning hair
- Hair loss
- Brittle hair that breaks easily
- Greying hair
- Oily hair

So, what can you do to support healthy hair throughout the years?

Your lifestyle plays a huge role in your hair health history and future. How well you nourish your body, hydrate your cells, supplement your system, rest your body, and destress your soul, all play a tremendous role in the hair you see and feel growing from within. Eating a whole-foods diet rich in plant-based nutrients, healthy sources of protein, ample fats, and fibre are essential. Supplementing with key nutrients such as antioxidants, phytonutrients, omegas, and collagen, and healing any specific and individual deficiencies you may have will make a world of a difference.

Become product educated and steer clear of chemical-based products that strip your hair of healthy oils and are full of xenoestrogens that impact your endocrine system, specifically your thyroid, reproductive system, and breast health. This is not only essential in your quest to healthy beautiful hair but also to your body as a whole.

Managing your level of stress is also key to support the right hormonal balance for healthy hair growth as well as your nails and skin. And sleep ladies—I cannot stress this über-important tip enough to you all. Sleep is the magic ingredient to the whole-body health you are after. It is where your body shifts into a state of "rest and digest"; otherwise known as your "parasympathetic nervous system." This is where our bodies unwind on every level and the real healing work within your brain and entire endocrine system begins to take place. Tapping into this system is critical for any health or healing goal you have. Honour your body and hormones by aiming to have your lights out by no later than 10 p.m. I know it sounds like a challenge, but I promise if you give it time you won't regret it. This is a core principle within all of my Women's Health and Hormone courses. Your entire body, including your hair, will thank you again and again.

As you can see, diet and lifestyle factors have a huge impact on hair health. The great news is that you can be in control of them if you choose. The question is, how badly you do you want healthy hair? What are you willing to give up to achieve the results you want for your hair?

Top Nutrients for Healthy Hair		
Nutrients	What They Do	Sources
Iron[18] Note: There are two types of iron, heme and non-heme. Heme iron comes from animal protein, and non-heme iron is found in plant-based foods. Heme iron is more easily absorbed by the body than non-heme iron.	When you don't have enough iron, your body can't produce the hemoglobin in your blood. Hemoglobin carries oxygen for the growth and repair of cells in your body, including the cells that stimulate hair growth. With treatment, you can help reverse both the iron deficiency and the hair loss.	*Heme iron foods:* Liver; Oysters, clams, and mussels; Red meats such as beef and lamb; Canned sardines; Chicken and turkey; Veal; Fish (Choose organic meats when possible) *Non-heme iron foods:* Beets; Cooked beans and lentils; Tofu; Pumpkin, squash, or sesame seeds; Chickpeas, kidney beans, and lima beans; Dried apricots; Baked potatoes; Nuts; Broccoli stems; Raw and cooked spinach and kale; Peas

Top Nutrients for Healthy Hair		
Zinc	Zinc plays an important role in hair tissue growth and repair. It also helps keep the oil glands around the follicles working properly. Hair loss is a common symptom of zinc deficiency.	Dark chocolate, nuts, seeds, legumes, shellfish, meat, eggs, whole grains
Vitamin B6 (pyridoxine) and B7 (biotin)[19]	Vitamin B6 helps the body make new red blood cells, which carry oxygen throughout the body. It also helps keep the immune system strong. Vitamin B7 is essential for healthy hair, nails, and nerve function	Whole grains (brown rice, barley, millet); Meat (red meat, poultry, fish); Eggs; Legumes (beans, lentils); Seeds and nuts (sunflower seeds, almonds); Dark green leafy vegetables (broccoli, spinach, kale); Fruits (citrus fruits, avocados, bananas)

Top Nutrients for Healthy Hair		
Omega-3 fatty acids[20]	Omega-3 fatty acids are essential and contribute to lubricating hair follicles and adding elasticity and brightness to your hair.	Fish and other seafood (especially cold-water fatty fish, such as salmon, mackerel, tuna, herring, and sardines); Nuts and seeds (such as flaxseed, chia seeds, pumpkin seeds, walnuts, and almonds); Plant oils: algal oil, flaxseed oil, avocado oil, sea buckhorn berry oil, raspberry seed oil, and tomato seed oil Tip #1: Refrigerate oils, nuts, and seeds so they don't oxidize and go rancid. Tip #2: Supplement with a plant-based omega such as Juice Plus+.

Top Nutrients for Healthy Hair		
Antioxidants	Antioxidants are molecules that fight free radicals in your body. Antioxidants neutralize free radicals to keep hair healthy and strong. Plant-based foods are rich in antioxidants.	A colourful plant-based diet: Fruits, berries, and green leafy vegetables Tip #1: The Environmental Working Group (EWG) has a list of the top 15 fruits and vegetables to buy without chemicals to reduce your toxic load. (See the resources section on page 235.) Tip #2: Add a whole-food plant concentrate, such as Juice Plus+ to your diet to bridge the gap.
Silica	Silica is an essential beauty mineral that helps heal brittle bones, teeth, hair, and nails.	Found in common vegetables such as onions, garlic, green leafy vegetables, carrots, cucumbers, and bell peppers, and in most sprouted seeds

Transitioning to Grey: Comments from My Grey-Hair Heroes

One of the things I love about social media and being a part of online groups is that you can pose questions on any topic and get feedback immediately. I have posed many questions to my Grey-Hair Heroes over the last year. Here I share with you a recent one that really grabbed my attention. I asked them to fill in the blank in the sentence: "I stopped colouring my hair and _____ improved." I received over two hundred comments. Here are some of them:

✓ Bank account
✓ Migraines gone
✓ Scalp improved; no more scaly patches
✓ I no longer get an itchy scalp and dye under my fingernails from scratching
✓ Hair loss is reversing
✓ Burning and itchy scalp gone
✓ Better self-esteem
✓ Psoriasis and rosacea cleared up
✓ My attitude
✓ State of mind
✓ Dry hair improved
✓ Constant sinus infections disappeared (this was from a hairstylist who changed careers)
✓ Skin health
✓ Security in who I am (once it grew out)
✓ I had a really bad rash on my chest and sometimes my neck on and off for a couple of years. I mistakenly thought it was caused by a food allergy or stress. When I stopped dying my hair the rash went away. That was fourteen months ago, and I haven't had that rash at all since.

✓ I no longer get hives or itchy lumps all over my scalp.

✓ Thyroid antibodies vanished

✓ Scabs on my scalp, burning on my head, night tremors, blood-pressure issues improved

✓ My skin improved, allergy gone. My hair texture improved, less dry and brittle

✓ No more scalp irritation, hair is thicker and not dry, no more dye on the bathroom walls, free time and money.

✓ The feeling of being the real me. And my hair is in great condition.

✓ Definitely my confidence and uplifted attitude. I felt so free knowing I gave myself permission to ditch the dye. I swear I was giddy.

✓ No more bald spots

✓ New hair growth

✓ I started a modelling career, who knew!

✓ Confidence! I always felt insecure about the "annoying" silver roots that would poke through a fresh dye job not even two weeks later! I felt like people were always looking at my roots. No more!

✓ My health, particularly my immune system! I've had autoimmune issues for a long time and I had a huge improvement. Also feeling authentic and confident!

✓ Gained precious time to spend other than sitting in salon for two hours every three weeks. Priceless

✓ Peace of mind

✓ My self-confidence. My hair is healthier and I get at least one compliment a day from a total stranger.

✓ Freedom

The comments I got from the question I posed had such an impact on me. They blew me away. The improvements were incredible, including better health and *hair*! Yeah! I had no idea so many women's lives would improve in so many areas because they stopped the dye. Goose bump moment! These comments were a reminder of why I wrote this book: To create a movement of women to ditch the dye for *better health*, a sense of *freedom* and *happiness*!

The dreaded *Grey Transition*: What to Do?

I spoke to Jalisa, a hairstylist at Altera Salon for over ten years, and this is what she had to say about hair today and her own experience:

It is very rare that I see healthy hair today in my salon. Most women today are bleaching or highlighting their hair, which can be very damaging to the hair over time. As women start to grey, they naturally want to start going lighter to have a better blend experience. Going from dark to blonde is the hardest transition and damages the hair the most. Every time we bleach the hair, we are pulling it apart and leaving it hollow, which makes the hair weak and massive breakage may occur. When women come in and ask how fast they can transition to *grey* or platinum blonde, and they have dark hair, they don't realize how long it's going to take without major damage to the hair. To prove this to my clients, I decided to go platinum blonde. My hair at the time was dyed *red*. I bleached it every day for one week straight to get the red out. I continued to bleach it in weeks two and three, and my hair turned orange. I waited two weeks before bleaching it again, which then left me with a burned scalp and painful puss bubbles. It took another two weeks for my scalp to heal before I started adding toner and colour. The condition of my hair was like straw and it had tons of breakage. This process took approximately one-and-a-half months before I had the results I wanted, which lasted about three weeks before the silver started to fade away, and then I was dealing with my natural dark roots. This transition takes time and money so women need to be prepared to see their hairdressers often if they don't have naturally grey roots. I regret doing this at the speed I did because I damaged my hair so much. From my personal experience, I can now talk honestly about the transition with clients and give them a reality check about what damage could happen to their hair. I warn you about all those pretty silver-haired models we see popping up everywhere, the truth is that there is a ton of Photoshopping going on—and blue light filters that can produce a very unrealistic image. If it's not natural, the upkeep of the trendy silver colour isn't realistic for most women.

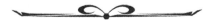

In October of 2018, I was thinking about letting my natural sparkle come through but I wasn't sure what the best path would be, so I did some research. I watched some YouTube videos and made a decision on what path I was going to take. The options I discovered might help you decide what would work best for you.

The Options

1. ***Shave your head:*** I honestly thought about this one as being the most simple and affordable way to just embrace the change. I also think it is the *bravest* option by far. Why? Because we are so attached to our hair and how it defines us. Imagine if we could get to that place of nonattachment and start all over again. It would be like a rebirth plus the temporary itchy scalp from the hair growth. I obviously was not ready to give birth again on that level. I know three women who took this path and who are in my Gorgeous Grey Movement (GGM) group on Facebook (see the resources section on page 235), and I have followed their journeys. They are the *bravest* women I know, and I'm so proud of them for making the choice. You will meet all three Brave Sparkle Heroes in the next chapter.

2. ***Grow out cold turkey:*** I also considered this path but lasted only about two months before I gave in to highlights. My long dark hair would show a white skunk line only after a week of dying my hair. I thought the process could move quickly, but I was wrong. The first two months were the hardest watching each day as my skunk line came into view. I estimated that it would take about five years to grow out based on how long my hair was, and the impatient me was not going to wait. I saw beautiful women on FB groups showing off this path, and I admired them from a distance, but I knew I wouldn't last this slow process.

3. ***Short pixie cut:*** This option is a popular one as it can be a fast transition of three to six months,

depending how short you go. I have seen great funky cuts that really compliment the face and natural colour. This is what my mom did when she turned fifty and decided to go grey. She got the short pixie cut and it grew out was fast and easily, which saved her time and money. She's had her grey pixie cut for almost seventeen years now, and it looks amazing on her. She has always added a splash of purple to the front to show off her bright playful personality. I had a pixie cut for so many years while raising young kids, and after four years of growing it out, I wasn't ready to cut it all off.

4. *Instant grey transformation:* I remember being on the edge of my seat when I watched a beauty blogger attempt to do this. She had long dark hair to her mid-back, and she wanted in one appointment to instantly be grey to match her natural colour. She had an all-day appointment, and the results would make any women drop to her knees and cry. She got the hair colour she wanted in a day, but she also lost half her hair (yes, it fell out by the handful), and she ended up getting a short bob. This was definitely not the path I was going to take. Too risky for me.

5. *Highlights:* The purpose of this option is to help you blend your sparkles in with your dyed hair. Depending on how dark your hair is, this could take a while and cost a lot for each foil treatment. If you already have lighter hair it would be a much easier process. With my dark hair, this is where I decided to start. It took about three

appointments to really start noticing a better blending experience, but I still wasn't happy with the look it was giving me; I wanted more.

6. ***Bleaching and toner:*** This option gives you better blending results; however, it comes with a cost. You need to invest in time, money, and patience with the risk of really damaging your hair. Guess what path I took. This one silly me! It took ten months of grow-out and about seven appointments of highlights, bleaching, toner, and colour to get to a full sparkle transition. I was every colour of hair as I was lightening it. I called it "rainbow hair" as I never really knew what colour I would leave with after a treatment. We went slowly to make sure we were protecting my hair and reducing the risk of breakage. Damaging the hair is going to happen. You can't avoid it when moving from dark hair to bleach blonde to grey. I had to cut off approximately eight inches of hair because there was so much damage, and it felt like straw. I also chose to use an organic salon and their products to reduce as many toxins as possible. My hair is now shoulder length, and I am more than half way to all my natural colour shining through. Yes, I got help from my hairdressers to move me more quickly to my natural sparkle, but I am really happy with the results. My hair isn't as damaged as it could be with all the extra love I gave it. I have had many hydrating treatments. I rarely use a dryer and only wash my hair once a week. Would I choose this path again if I could start all over? Not sure! I have calculated that I have spent about twenty-four

hours of my life in the last ten months in a salon working on my hair, plus over $1,500 investing in this transition, all in the name of vanity. I am hoping this transition stage is over and I can enjoy my natural sparkle forever.

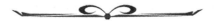

I chose Jalisa as my hairstylist to finish my transition to silver because she had her own personal experience and helped others successfully transition. She warned me that it was going to be approximately a seven-hour appointment, which I didn't believe. I joked with her and said, "You can do it in five, right?" Nope, it took seven and a half hours! Just to be clear, I had already had six appointments over ten months slowly transitioning to a better blend experience. This last appointment was going to be the longest by far, and it was built on seventeen hours of salon work before we could do this final step. Jalisa had to foil every piece of hair that was not natural grey, then bleach it out, tone it, wash it, foil it again with up to six different grey/silver colours to match my natural colour. The final result was a perfect blend to my natural sparkle, and I would say it was worth it. I guess that I'm ten to twelve months away from my hair being fully grown out if I keep it at shoulder length. I sped up the process and I'm happy with the results. I have such a new appreciation to hair colourists and the work they create. It truly is a science. No turning back, just patience now. Whatever you decide is the best path for you is perfectly okay! And if you're worried about what people think, it's none of their business! The only person who matters in this transition is *you*!

So now that you have grey natural hair, how do you keep it healthy? I posed this question to some hairstylist friends. They agreed that natural grey strands have a tendency to frizz and can easily look dull if you don't keep up. Here were some of their tips to keeping your grey hair polished:

1. Don't forget UV protection. Since grey hair lacks pigment, it can easily be tinted by external factors such as fluorescent lights, the sun, styling heat products, and even pollution. They recommend using a spritz-on UV protectant, especially in the summer months.

2. Use a clarifying shampoo once a week to help remove unwanted buildup on your hair, which can occur from hard water and styling products. This will keep your grey hair shiny. An affordable way to do this at home with no chemicals is to use apple cider vinegar. Apple cider vinegar will stimulate your hair follicles and clean clogged pores. How do I use this home remedy?
   - Mix a couple of tablespoons of apple cider vinegar with water.
   - Add a few drops of your favourite essential oil (e.g., lavender).
   - After shampooing and conditioning, pour the mixture evenly over your hair, working it into your scalp.
   - Let it sit for a couple of minutes.
   - Rinse it out.
   - Results: Clean hair.

3. Try purple products to counteract yellow tones that can pop up in the grey strands. If your hair takes on a violet cast consider trying a blue-hued

shampoo and conditioner a few times a month. My hair seems to take on a yellowish cast, so they suggested lathering a couple times a month with a silver-specific shampoo. My personal experience is that you have to play a bit with different shampoos because some can really change your colour; don't panic, it's just temporary. That purple cast will rinse out in your next shower when you use your regular shampoo. I am currently using the Organic ColourSystems Purple Shampoo and Conditioner which seems to be working well. (See the resources section on page 235.)

4. Get a trim every six to eight weeks to keep clean edges. Grey hair can start to look unruly if it's not trimmed enough. Make sure your stylist doesn't use a razor because it can cause the ends to fray, making it seem out of control.

5. Add a hair mask at least once a month to help improve hydration, increase shine, and reduce frizz. You can purchase a hair mask at your favourite salon or retail store, or ask your stylist for a treatment next time you're at the salon. Read your labels and find one that has a clean ingredient list. If you want to save money, you can consider using some basic kitchen items to create your own hair mask. This is my home remedy hair mask: 1 tablespoon (15 mL) of coconut oil, 1 tablespoon (15 mL) of honey, and half avocado. Mash them all together and rub into your hair. Leave it on for at least twenty minutes, and then rinse it out with warm water. Your hair will feel and look amazing.

As you have learned, healthy hair is more than just popping a magic pill and slathering some oil on it. Healthy hair starts with what you feed your body and your lifestyle factors. Our hair goes through cycles as our bodies change and our hormones fluctuate. We need to show patience and compassion when we go through these changes and adapt accordingly. Eventually for most of us, our hair will start to turn grey at some point (a worldwide study showed that between 45 and 65 years of age, 74% of people were affected by grey hair[21]), and we will need to decide what path we will take: to embrace it or to dye it. Whatever you decide, may you continue to be inspired to go for *healthy hair*!

CHAPTER SEVEN

Sparkle Stories from the Heart

"We are all stars and we deserve to twinkle."
—MARILYN MONROE

We all deserve to shine bright in this world. This chapter is all about the brave ones who have gone before me or who have joined me on the sparkle journey. Who doesn't like a good story? A story that inspires. A story that makes you cry. I have always been drawn to people's stories. I grew up with a love for watching documentaries and reading biographies as I got older. The story. Hearing someone's heart, their struggles, their breakthroughs and the "aha" moment that changed their path. I have hand-picked some amazing women from my Gorgeous Grey Movement (GGM) Facebook group to share their hearts and learn how they became brave enough to let their grey sparkle shine through. Thank you, my brave friends for sharing your hearts and inspiring others to consider ditching the dye.

I gave my GGM women six questions to answer:
1. When did you first start to colour your hair? Why? (How old were you?)

2. Why did you decide it was time to let your grey/white/silver sparkle? (How old were you?)

3. What did you do to transition to grey? (i.e., shave, pixie, highlights, bleach to blend, let it go naturally)

4. Going grey can be very emotional. Negative comments, dreaded skunk line, and fear of the unknown. What was the transition like for you?

5. How do you feel about your grey hair today?

6. Do you have any advice for women who are thinking about joining the Gorgeous Grey Movement?

Sparkle Stories from the Heart
Janice Neigum: My mom, my hero, my mentor
Age: 67
Alberta, Canada

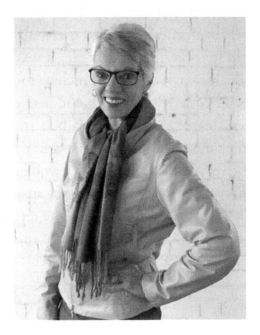

1. I first started colouring my hair as a teen at fourteen; it was *the* thing to do. I didn't dye my hair often, just now and again for fun. I started colouring seriously in my forties as I was showing lots of grey.
2. In 2005, at the age of fifty-three, I did a month-long detox, and from then on I became more conscious of health and toxins. I used henna dyes from then on when I worked in the health-food store in the summer of 2005. I decided that after my son Josh's wedding in October 2006 I had had enough of covering up my greys.
3. As I transitioned, I just kept getting my hair cut, it was challenging, but I was persistent.

4. My husband was my biggest fan as he thought women with grey hair looked hot. I did hear some negative comments, but I never let that change how I felt about going grey. It was freedom to not have to dye my hair and cover up to look younger or to fit in with the social norms.

5. Today I feel comfortable with my grey hair, and I love to put a purple sparkle in the front. It's a washable colour, so I get to decide each day how much to rock my purple.

6. The Gorgeous Grey Movement is the perfect social place to feel loved, learn great tips, and be surrounded with empowered women who will support your decision. It is so interesting to see all the beautiful, grey women and hear the vast opinions of so many beautiful, grey sparklers! I am so proud of the decision Nicole made to go grey, and I admire her vision to create a safe and fun place to support other women on the journey. Get your Silver Fox on and feel the freedom!

Roxanne Piche
Age: 60
Saskatchewan, Canada

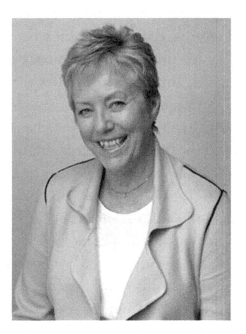

1. I started colouring my hair when I was in my twenties, so that would be about forty years of home colours (not so great), to salon appointments (very expensive), to bring me back to the blonde that I was so used to when I was younger.

2. I decided to own my sparkle about two-and-a-half years ago. I was in a tight financial position paying off debt, and the cost of my salon appointments was too much. I would have been in my late fifties when I decided to let my natural colour grow out.

3. I have short hair, but always had highlights done to blend in the noticeable grey hairs that were present, especially around my face. It was time to let it go natural.

4. At the time and it still is, that grey became the new blonde, and the younger generation were dying their hair to look like mine! So it really was an easy decision on my part to stop dying it. There was a transition phase, where the blonde had to grow out to the point where I could cut it off, but I was determined not to go back to the route of highlighting it again, and within a few months and after a good cut, it was gone.

5. Now I love my sparkle. It's more silver/white than a hard grey, and the back is still darker than silver, but I'm looking forward to owning a glorious head of full white hair!

6. I own it, it's mine, and I am proud to be a woman of age and not be pressured to be or look like someone I'm not! Why do we, at any age, allow others' opinions of us define who we are? If family or friends are criticizing you for making the decision to grow out your grey, then ask them to pay for your salon appointment and see how fast they shut up! Listen to your own opinion and what matters to you as a woman first. Transition at your own pace and own who you are at any age! Proud Member of the Gorgeous Grey Movement!

Andrea Munro White

Age: 44

Ontario Canada

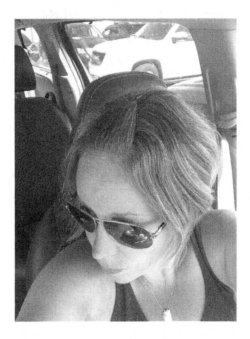

1. I was nineteen and I got a gift certificate for Christmas. I just wanted a different look. I thought my hair was dull looking and, if I'm honest, it was *the thing* to do.

2. I was forty-three when I decided it was time to "sparkle." I had wanted to for almost a year but didn't have the courage and I talked myself out of it until Nicole started this movement. It was just the push I needed. Confidence in numbers, right?

3. Once I decided to let my "sparkle shine," my hairdresser decided to put toner in my hair to help blend the blonde highlights I already had. We first did a blunt cut, and then I went for it and had it cut really short on the back and sides with some length at the front so I still felt feminine.

4. The transition for me in terms of acceptance was seamless. Once I decide to do something, I just go for it. No opinions or comments sway me. Besides, my husband loves it, my kids think it's cool, and the other comments that I've received have no emotional impact. If anything, they give me a laugh. I do wish the grow-out process would be faster though.

5. I'm still in the process of transitioning to my grey. I still have a ways to go. I'm loving what I see so far. The most shocking is the grey that's revealing itself. I've been dying my hair for so long I didn't realize how much sparkle I really had. It is hard to envision what it will look like when it's done, but I can't wait to see myself in all *my own* sparkle!

6. My advice is simple: To those who are considering to "own their own sparkle," the hardest part is making the decision to "sparkle," but once you decide you are ready to do it, own it and just go for it! Enjoy and be open to the journey. Just be careful of the confidence you'll get from owning it!

Christine Ransome-Mcconkey

Age 57
Alberta, Canada

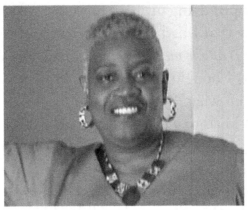

1. I was forty-two years old. I did it out of vanity. I believed that if I let my hair grey, then I would look old. In addition, my hairdresser loved to encourage me to try different colours. As for my friends, they all dye their hair, so I felt a lot of peer pressure to dye my hair as well.

2. I stopped at age fifty-five. Reason: I was getting too obsessed with wanting to cover the grey, and I was dying my hair every two weeks. But the major reason I stopped was that the chemicals started to negatively affect me. The strong chemicals were causing pimples on my scalp; my scalp was tingling and eventually that tingling expanded down my arms to my fingers! The smell of the dyes was also affecting me. I realized I had to stop exposing myself to those chemicals.

3. I cut it all off and bought a wig to let my natural hair grow out. Once it grew, I could then style it. I was very self-conscious at first and I didn't own it. I wore the wig every time I stepped outside my house. Then gradually I decided to go to the mall once a week without the wig.

This was a *huge* step for me. To my surprise, I bumped into some friends, they saw my new sparkle, and they complimented me. Some of my close friends were happy that I stopped dying my hair; however, a few friends were not happy that I had gone grey. To those friends, I told them *this is about me, not you*. To make myself feel more confident, I bought big hoop earrings and always wore my makeup when I went out.

4. I realized I had to *own* it and carry my head high. It was difficult in the beginning because I was so self-conscious and worried about what others may say or think and how they might react.

5. During the transition with old dyed hair and new grey hair, I used a "grey shampoo," which prevented me from getting that washed-out yellowing or blueish colour as the dyed hair grew out. Today I feel fabulous, and going grey was very *freeing* for me. I remind myself that I am doing this for *me*, not my spouse or friends.

6. I encourage other women to do it; it's a natural process, so why fight it. You need to enjoy it. *Just do it*! It's a *free* feeling—freedom from chemicals. *Embrace* your new-found freedom!

Pamela Sue
Age: 64
Hawaii, USA

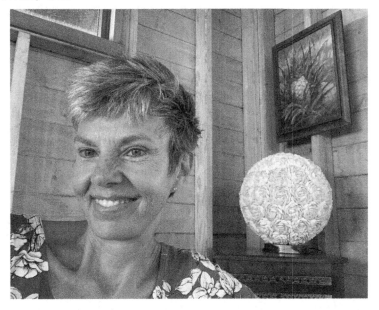

1. In 1998 I was in my forties, was experiencing health challenges, and my hair looked terrible. I didn't want to add to the toxicity I was battling by colouring my hair, and then I found Aveda's concept for hair colour derived from plant essences that were much less toxic. I took the plunge and was very happy *until* the grey roots starting showing up more and more prominently.

2. I had been wanting to do it for quite a few years because colouring the roots was not an enjoyable experience month after month, but I was always talked out of it, especially by my hairdressers. The only process that made sense to me was to cut it all off and start over. I had cut all my hair off once before, and the growing-out process was very painful. I was avoiding what I knew I'd have to experience. I finally just got sick and tired of being sick and tired of

those roots showing up every month and saw so many other women with grey hair who looked gorgeous, and after talking with them over the years, I finally decided it was *time*. I did it in time for my birthday—next month I'll be sixty-four.

3. Shave it all off! I knew once I decided to do it, that that was what I'd do. I don't have the patience for any other options.

4. I don't really care what people think, so that wasn't an issue for me, although it was an act of courage to make such a drastic change to let go of two pounds of hair! I had to find the guts, knowing I'd have to go through that painful growing out experience again. But timing is everything and it was time! I must say I was surprised by a friend who was opposed to my plan and got emotional over my decision; that friend was very attached to my hair. It was amazing to me that this would affect someone else that profoundly. I immediately posted my pictures on social media and was surprised at the support. I guess those who didn't like it kept their comments to themselves. That was one way to capture attention.

5. I'm not sure why it took me so long other than that I just wasn't ready. I'm not sure if I'll like my hair grey or not. But I do know that I was tired of going through the "roots process" month after month, and I will never go back to that process with my hair. However, I do appreciate *wig technology* and will embrace that while I'm going through the painful "grow-out." I've always been a fan of Dolly Parton, and she *never* tries to hide her age and will tell people how long she's been married to her husband (over fifty years!). I don't want to hide my age either and never have, although I completely agree with Dolly when she says, "If something

is sagging, dragging, or bagging I'll get nipped, tucked or sucked." Dolly doesn't do those things because she is trying to hide her age, she does them because she doesn't like the way they make her look and feel, and she can afford to fix it! Why not? If I like the way wigs look and feel, I might just stick with those, who knows? But I'll do it because that is what I want to do, not because I'm trying to be someone or an age I'm not. I'm proud to be sixty-four, and I'll do my best to feel my best, to be and look the best I can be, but I know the days of dying my hair are over! And it feels *great* to have finally taken that step!

6. It has been six months since I made the decision to "go grey." For ten years I had suffered with monthly migraine headaches. I don't know why it never occurred to me that saturating my head with chemicals for thirty minutes every month could be a cause for this monthly debilitation, but apparently it was. Stopping the colour is the only thing I changed; it's been six months now, and I have yet to experience a migraine! To me this is a miracle and true beauty truly comes from within!

Do it for *you* not anyone else. If it's your desire and you see women who have done it and you admire their look, tell them! Ask questions, listen to them, how long ago did they do it? How do they feel about it now? I don't think I've ever heard anyone say they regretted it, but how would we know? If they did regret it, we wouldn't see them because maybe they went back to colouring. And that is an option we have if we want to. It's *just hair*, and you know what, it grows back! Take your time making your decision, don't rush into it. Be sure it's right for you. Know this is another opportunity for personal transformation and growth—to be brave and courageous and true to yourself.

April Wooley
Age: 56
Ontario, Canada

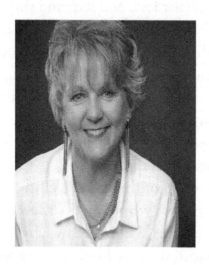

1. My first introduction to hair dye was a product called Sun In. It was used when you were outside in the sun, and active while swimming, or not. The general idea was to spray it onto your hair and it would gradually bleach it. I started using it on summer vacations at the family cottage. The usual reason: advertising led me to believe that I was "cooler" and more attractive as I sported blonde streaks. Sun-kissed hair and skin was a sign of health and wealth in the 1970s.

2. I decided to "sparkle" by embracing my grey hair because I perceived "showing your roots" to be trashy. When a woman showed her roots, I equated it as an indicator that she didn't care about herself. I believe I was around thirty to thirty-five when I started experimenting with letting my grey hair emerge. It was difficult at first because of texture change and varying shades of brown, which was my original colour. It was a dull look, so I kept it short.

3. The transition: I continued keeping it short as the brown and grey attempted to play well together. For the first year and a bit, it remained dull looking. I found that oil-based haircare products gave my hair a healthier appearance. I found that dying was expensive, and I was done dying. I decided to let the grey come in.

4. Emotions: I don't recall any personal negativity. However, there were comments such as, "Your husband's going to be looking for a younger woman," and "People are going to think you're twice your age." Comments like that. During the transition I remember wearing makeup more often, and applying it a number of times during the day. Particularly lipstick. Probably an attempt to distract attention away from my hair.

5. Today: I cherish it. I have been full-on grey for about twenty-nine years now! By far one of the best decisions I ever made. When I reflect back, I received compliments all the time. At least twice a week. People, men and women, would tell me how great it is. How it suits me. And these are people I don't even know. My grey hair can be fun, sexy, intimidating, empowering—separately or all at once. I can honestly say that I will never return to dying my hair. I've earned and learned so much. There is a peacefulness that grey hair provides. It's a validation of my authenticity. A badge of honour if you will. My grey hair says, "I've arrived."

6. Advice: Do it! Approach it as giving yourself the best gift ever. The gift that keeps on giving. Every time you see it, touch it. Envision it as your reality. Slow steps. It can take time. Emotional time to transition. The transition time will come with challenges, usually from others as careless remarks. That's okay. View the challenges as

opportunities to grow. I believe you grow in confidence, patience, and inner strength. Some people in your close circle will see your grey hair as a threat. Subconsciously they know you are owning yourself, and sometimes that makes people nervous.

Angela Horne
Age: 55
Ontario Canada

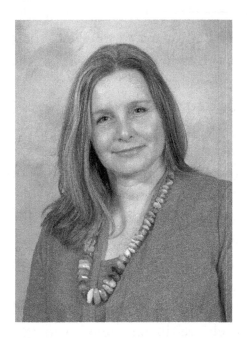

1. I remember I first started to colour my hair for fun in my late twenties, and then I felt the need to let my natural colour, which was chestnut brown, come in. About six weeks later, I started to notice a few strands of sparkles starting to find their way through.

2. At age thirty-five, I started to feel peer pressure to colour my hair to cover up the sparkle. I had noticed over a few years that I was colouring more, and I had never been a high-maintenance girl. By the age of forty-six my hair truly became part of a regular maintenance routine and it wasn't fun anymore. It was becoming too much work. I found that the more I tried to colour my hair brown, the lighter it became and turned into a light blonde. My hair was trying to tell me to go light and let all the sparkle

shine through, and so my journey of growing my hair began.

3. I guess I can say I was lucky because my hair was rebelling and it was turning lighter and not holding the colour, so the transition for me was easier. I did go for a really good cut and had low lights put in so the silver started to appear as highlights.

4. I had received some not-so-favourable comments about why I was letting my grey hair grow, "You look so much prettier with darker hair." The other was, "Oh, you're growing into an old lady now, huh?" Another comment was, "Oh, you aren't going to like it at all," or "Your hair is going to be so wiry and will lose its shine and be dull and greasy."

5. I had regular trimmings for the new growth, which I found to make it a healthy transition. The more I let my hair grow, the more it felt stronger and healthier. The full process to achieve the outcome I wanted to achieve was about two years, and that was manageable.

6. I just knew in my heart it was time and the right choice for me. I was seeing more and more pictures of beautiful women with long sassy sparkle hair, and I was excited for the new me who was emerging right before my eyes. I also made a vow to love myself and the process, no matter what because inside I am beautiful, and this is what I see. My final thought regarding going forward is that if it feels good inside, do it on the outside. Love who you are today!

Jineen Glover
Age: 44
Texas, USA

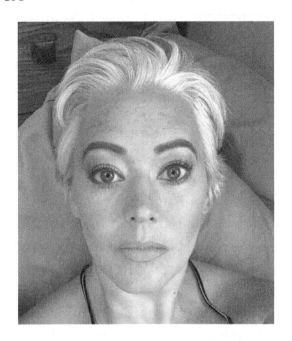

1. I first started colouring my hair in college. I coloured it mostly for a certain look, but I also had a few grey hairs starting in my early twenties.

2. I had always wanted to shave my head as a bucket-list thing, and when my niece was diagnosed with Hodgkin's lymphoma, I thought I would shave my head for her to try to encourage her to realize that her hair wouldn't define her beauty. I had five weeks of root growth that I was covering up and decided to see what the colour would be like once my head was shaved. I also felt a nudge from God to go for it. I felt that it could be life changing for me. I've always appreciated authenticity and desired to be authentic, and it felt as though this was another way in which I could really live my authentic and true self. I was

wanting to let go of what society said about hair colour, beauty, and aging. I wanted to be a part of redefining beauty. It really was a letting go of so many things for me when I shaved my head. I was forty-three when I did this.

3. The transition has been interesting for me. I have received so many compliments, so that is nice, but I definitely have had to adjust to the new me.

4. I've missed my dark-brown hair since I was always a brunette, and then because I shaved it off, I just missed my hair! It was more than one adjustment. I do think I went through a bit of a grieving process over the loss of my hair, and feeling the loss of my hair colour and the identity of who I had been. I was mostly concerned that I was now going to look old, but I think the silver actually softened me.

5. Today, after almost six months on this journey, I like my hair more as it has grown out and the colour seems to get prettier and prettier! I have to say it has been a relief to not have to dye my hair every two weeks, and I actually have more hair and healthier hair now!

6. The only advice I can give is to do what your heart is telling you to do. Let go of the stigma that people once had about grey hair. It is just another colour, and it is so freeing to really be authentically you and not negatively influenced by society. Do it when you are ready to surrender and let go!

Nikki Cotton
Age: 69
USA

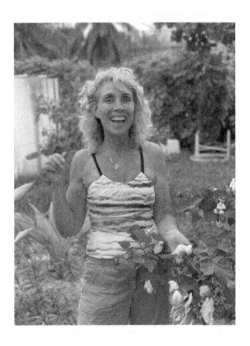

1. Honestly, I can't remember when I started colouring my hair. I do remember I bought home colouring kits and just did my whole head as close to the colour that my natural colour was, maybe in my mid-forties. I had my daughters when I was thirty-six and thirty-nine years old. As they began to dance and play sports, I found myself on the field or in the studio with moms who were often ten years younger than I was. They always guessed me to be close to their age, and I loved that they thought I was younger than I actually was. Fascinating to me now, the importance of people's judging that you are younger than your chronological age! The solid dark colour, without highlights was not flattering, and as the grey came in more heavily, I started to get highlights and dye the roots! I am

not a spa person or a nail person, so I never enjoyed the process. It wasn't about being pampered; it was simply quick vanity that needed to be dealt with!

2. January 2016, I declared my new me and went grey/silver. (I still have a hard time saying grey, it feels flat and silver feels glitzy!) I was sixty-six years old and was tired of having to dye the dreaded slunk line every three weeks. For the previous two years I had asked my hairdresser, *every time*, "Do you think I should go grey? Will I look older? How do we know if it will be the "good" grey?" And for those two years she said, "You'll look great and the colour is great."

3. Finally I said do it! I had no idea that I would walk out as a blonde! I have always had this weird idea that if I were to become blonde, I would be a traitor. Big judgment around all those brunettes who thought they would have "more fun" if they were blonde. So I left the salon as a "traitor." And every time someone commented, "Oh, I see you went blonde," my immediate and *bold* response was, "I am *not* going blonde, I am in transition." As my roots grew out, we began to tone the blonde and move into "silver." It didn't feel like a huge transition, just dealing with making sure people didn't think I was a blonde! Within a year I started loving my hair as the blonde disappeared and my natural grey was shining.

4. When I was contemplating it, I asked every grey-haired woman in every store how they made their transition, and let them know how brave I thought they were. I now have women come to me and ask me the same question. They complement me and tell me I am inspiring.

5. I *love* my colour! I think I look younger, more vibrant, and more natural. In fact, when I look at pictures of me with my dark hair, it looks as though I am wearing a wig!

6. My advice, don't bother colouring, let it come in naturally, enjoy each strand of silver woven in with your own colour, like the evolution of your wisdom, matching the rhythm of our lives, like a tapestry, ever changing. Let it represent your innate wisdom coming forth.

Heidi Biggs
Age: 47
From Hastings, England, to Santa Barbara, CA in 2005, to
Ventura County, CA

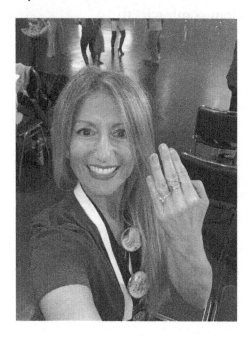

1. I first started colouring my hair when I was quite young,
   thirteen, I think. I had my fringe/bangs highlighted
   (my hair at that time was past my butt!), and I thought
   it was the best thing ever! Then after that I would buy
   a semi-permanent mahogany colour and put that on all
   over, it was the eighties and a very popular colour! I also
   knew when I was four that I would be a hairstylist. I was
   fourteen when I found my first grey hair—in my eyebrow
   of all places!

2. I was forty-six when I decided that I wanted to embrace
   my sparkle and let it shine. I decided that it was the best
   thing for me to do because every time I coloured my hair
   my favourite blonde, the grey strands at the front were

my favourite, giving me the confidence to say *yes*, I will love my grey hair. It just made sense!

3. The transition was easy, especially being a hairstylist. I just did with my own hair what I had previously done with my clients. Highlights toned silver to blend. I also added silver and blonde hair extensions. I have a plan! Leave the extensions in for a while, then once my white has grown out more, I will chop it into a bob and then grow it long but natural.

4. The transition truly has been easy, except the old stinking thinking that white hair makes you feel old! I would take a good long hard look at myself in the mirror and take notice of all of the things I loved about myself and then remembered white does not define your age, it is just purely and simply a colour, a colour that I actually love!

5. It was very interesting what others have said. I have had colleagues say negative things, and yet others be extremely supportive. I receive the most compliments from men, young women, and women my own age who wish they were confident enough to do the same. I simply tell them, you can! I simply love my white hair, and I can truly say I wish there was more of it! I cannot wait for the remaining dark hair to go.

6. I would encourage any woman or man to go for it and embrace the natural process. It is so empowering and liberating and just simply *fun*! If you are on the fence, I say, "What have you got to lose?" If you have fear surrounding doing it because you are afraid of what other people think, I say *#&$ what they think, do what you want for a change!

Anastasia Stambulski Takeda
Age: 57
Ontario Canada

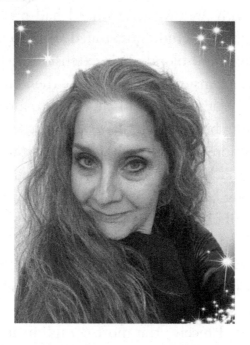

1. I started colouring my hair with highlights when I was in my twenties. As to why I started, hmm, trying to think back, I believe I did it for fun, for a change, something different right along with getting a new haircut or style.

2. Letting my grey sparkle was just something that evolved for me. In the past four to five years I had started using organic colour for low lights and highlights. I would only do it every six months to a year as I didn't have a definitive line with hair growth. It would just blend with the grey that had started coming in, and I didn't mind. I never had the desire to cover the grey completely. Life evolves and changes as do we, and likewise so does our hair.

3. Transitioning to grey was easy as I did highlights. It's a great way to blend while avoiding the harsh line that occurs with all-over colour.

4. It's important to be happy with who you are and realize that life is about constant change. Nothing stays the same. Change can be wonderful!

5. I love my grey hair today! It's part of who I am.

6. My advice to any woman or man thinking of joining the Gorgeous Grey Movement is go for it! Be confident and love who you are. You need to feel good about yourself in order to exude and spread positivity, love, and acceptance in this world. Let's make this wonderful movement viral!

Diane Pippi Marlene Karlyn
Age: 49
California, USA

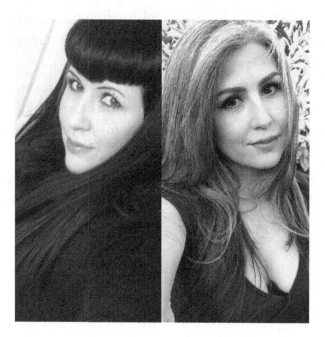

1. I was fifteen when I started to colour my hair. My mom
    gave me permission to dye my hair as long as the colour
    was similar to my natural brunette colour. I had no grey
    hair yet.

2. It was 2009/2010. I was thirty-nine/forty years old (I'm
    currently forty-nine). At that age, I already had quite a
    bit of silver roots showing, and I always coloured my
    hair to cover it up. I was inspired by the Pinterest posts
    of natural silver-haired women.

3. I didn't want that dreaded demarcation line, so I
    grew out parts of my silver first; for a year I grew out
    the bottom layer of my fringe/bangs and everything
    underneath. I continued to colour the crown of my
    head and the top layer of my fringe/bangs. In 2011, I

stopped colouring altogether and let nature fill in the silver!

4. The transition was quite smooth. Growing out portions for the first year really made the rest of the transition look seamless. It looked edgy and purposely coloured. I didn't receive any negativity from friends or family. I was very vocal about my plans to grow it out.

5. I love my grey hair so much. I love the colour pattern, the highlights of the silver, the lowlights of the grey. It's Mother Nature that gave me beautiful long silver streaks along my temples, fringe/bangs. When I get bored with my hair, I simply use temporary colours. So far, my hair has been blue and currently it's pink! It rinses out in a few weeks.

6. My advice would be to go for it! Whatever way you decide to, cold turkey, just stop colouring and go for it; chop it all off and have a hair rebirth; have a colourist bleach it out and use grey dyes or toners—whichever way that makes the transition comfortable. I love how big this movement is growing. I fully support women embracing what Mother Nature has given them. I also advise women to compliment other women and men they come across in their day-to-day lives. I compliment so many women with beautiful silver and grey hair who I see in public. I also receive lots of compliments from all age groups. I've also had my picture taken! I just want other women to be encouraged to continue to show their beautiful silver streaks.

Deb Lunney
Age 65
Ontario, Canada

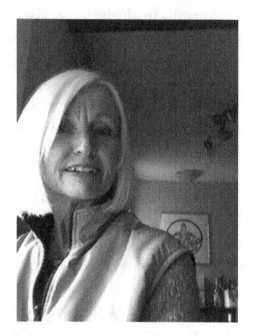

1. I started colouring my hair at age twenty-eight with henna to cover the grey. While in university, I had streaked my hair for highlights.

2. I let my hair go grey initially in my early forties, but went back to colour until I was fifty-two. I transitioned for a few reasons. I hated wasting two-hundred dollars every six weeks when roots would show long before the six-week mark. I also hated wasting the time at the hairdresser's, sitting there for two hours with a black cape on looking dreadful. One day while sitting in the chair, I was reading a novel, *Catcher in the Rye*, whose protagonist hated phoniness, and I thought that dying my hair at this point wasn't very authentic or true to myself.

3. I bleached my hair very light and let it grow in as much as possible, hid away for the summer at my cottage, and before returning to school in the fall, I cut my hair very short. My kids freaked out.

4. I remember going to the dentist in my forties just before my first "grow in," and they asked the usual question: "Any chance of pregnancy before x-rays?" However, six months later when I returned to dentist with grey hair, they asked me a new question: "Do you have any heart problems?" Interesting how quickly the question can change based on hair colour.

5. I'm happy to have my natural colour—white—today.

6. My advice is to avoid the toxins when you can. Avoiding colouring your hair is one way to protect your health, save time and money, and be natural.

Sahar Younes
Age: 52
Ontario, Canada

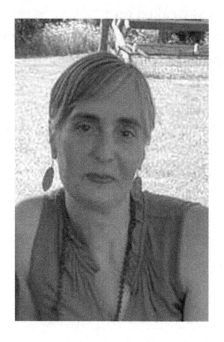

1. I started colouring at age thirty-one. I had never coloured before so it was only for grey cover that I started.

2. To reduce my exposure to toxins, I began using Herbatint around 2012. Although it was the less toxic option, the colour faded quickly and my grey would bleed through within a couple of weeks. For about two years I was colouring every two to three weeks and started contemplating just letting it go. My husband and kids actually said go for it, but my three sisters were all against it. I decided to do it anyway. Once I made the decision, my youngest sister came around and gave me some good advice, "Make sure you start wearing more colour," (I was a mostly black- and grey-clothing kind of girl), "and wear some makeup and earrings to ensure you don't look

or feel 'frumpy.'" My thought was that it wasn't forever and if I wasn't comfortable, I could just start colouring again.

3. I got it cut quite short and just waited to see what would happen.

4. The transition has been easy. I never experienced the skunk line as the Herbatint tended to fade rather than grow out. I feel fortunate that my silver grey is mostly in the front and looks like it's been highlighted that way. The rest of my hair isn't my youthful light-brown colour, but a darker grey, and it seemed to transition seamlessly over the year or so. I've had mixed reviews on my hair; a few people who hadn't seen me in a while were a bit shocked, and I got a few comments about "letting myself go," but it didn't bother me.

5. I love my hair! It's all in the attitude and presentation. I do make sure I've got lipstick and a little blush on when I'm out because I'm a bit pale, and with my hair there's not a lot of contrast. I also make sure I wear colours and nice earrings. Going grey actually made me more conscious of being stylish! I've never had an issue with my age and growing older, so maybe that's part of it.

6. Just do it! It really is in your perspective and attitude. Realize that your age means you have lived, loved and have much too offer. I saw a quote about our grey should be called *wisdom highlights* and I love that.

Martha Neigum (my bonus Grandma)
Age: 85
Alberta, Canada

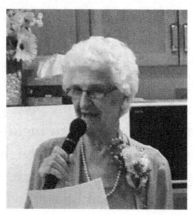

1. I was around forty when I started to dye my hair. A friend of mine talked me into colouring my hair. I continued to colour it and liked that I wasn't going to look older than I was.
2. I coloured for forty years and played around with different colours. I used a combination of hair-salon and home dyes.
3. I let my natural colour come in when I was eighty years old. Many of my friends and family already had gone grey, so I thought it was time and I finally felt ready.
4. My transition was easy, I just stopped colouring it and let my natural colour come in. My hair was short and natural curly, so it didn't take long to fully transition—less than six months.
5. I feel good about my new look, and I get many compliments as it is pure white. The bonus is, it is really health.
6. My advice: let your grey, or in my case white, hair come in when you are ready. I wasn't ready until I was eighty years old.

Pamela Ollenberger
Age: 46
Alberta, Canada

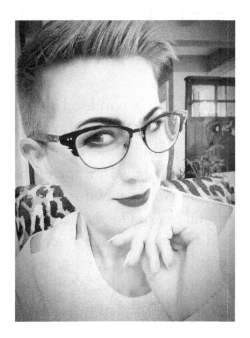

1. I started to dye my hair at age of 37 I believe. Why? I wanted to be a woman who didn't look old as society shames us from being gray and looking nothing than youthful and vibrant. I was in a lackluster marriage, trying to be someone I was not. Many times as women we color our hair for reasons that are below the surface and only tell others we are doing it to "look good" which is often a lie.
2. I am turning 46 in August and I decided to stop fighting myself. I came to terms with my age and my life. I was for once happy and in love with my soulmate/twin flame.
3. On a whim I shaved my hair and colored it silver. That day I felt alive at the salon, knowing *this is it*!
4. The transition made me feel in control, excited, nervous, scared - every emotion one could feel, I felt. I had so

much gray hair feathering through my sides and crown area that I just didn't want to color it and be someone I was fighting to become. This was a profound opportunity for self-acceptance and making peace with myself as an aging woman. I have received lots of compliments since making the change, and others say they love it more! Imagine that.

5. I feel liberated, free, and happy. I feel like I can accomplish anything now. I feel like the woman I was meant to become. I don't need to hide anymore.

6. The advice I would share with women who are thinking about joining the Gorgeous Grey Movement is to not hesitate. Love and be kind to yourself. Stop fighting what is natural and become your best version of you. Find a hairstyle that is funky, fun, edgy and compliment it with your transition like I did. My life is full and I live an abundant life now with less material things that don't own me anymore. I now have a few very best friends and the most amazing lover who makes me feel appreciated and valued each and every day. Change is good!

Nicole Scott, Founder of the Gorgeous Grey Movement
Age: 48
Ontario, Canada

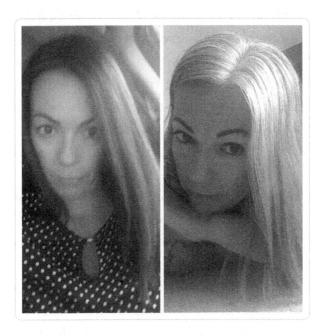

1. I started dying my hair in my teens. In grade 9 I took a beauty class (yes that was a thing in the eighties) and learned how to perm and dye hair. I realized very quickly I was not cut out for a career in hair, just ask my mom. I mostly did home dye jobs with different colors, as that was the cheapest option.

2. I noticed grey hair showing up in my twenties, and it started to really show up in my thirties. I wanted to stop dying by my mid-thirties after I took a course on nutrition. This is when I learned of the dangers of toxins in our beauty products. I got the nudge to stop dying from Spirit, and to write a book about it, but I wasn't ready! I continued to dye my hair until October 2018, when I finally made a decision after a health scare woke me up.

3. How was I going to transition to grey? I did a lot of research to figure out what felt right for me, and I decided to highlight and eventually bleach out my dark hair for a better blending experience. I was clear that I was done with root touch-ups forever, so the rule was: don't touch my roots, let them grow out naturally. I found an organic salon to help me with the transition to reduce the toxic load, which made a big difference in my symptoms. Looking back now, if I was to do it all over I would just have shaved it off and donated my hair to cancer but I was too afraid.

4. My transition was drastic because I had dark hair and my skunk line was noticeable at week two. After two months, I got highlights to start blending it better, but it took many trips to the salon, only to find a very expensive bill at the end of it. The first four months were hard—I'm not going to lie. After it started blending better, I started to really get excited. It gave me hope that I could do this. I did get a negative comment from a guy about three months in, asking, "Are you letting yourself go?" Well, my response was, "F*** you, if you can do it, why can't I?" I was pissed. This happened at a Christmas party, and it got to me so I left right then. What pissed me off the most was that he was grey and it was a double standard going on. I let it go and made it my motivation not to give in to one person making a negative comment. I needed to be strong to break this stereotype that has existed for far too long. I wanted to be part of the solution and an inspiration to others and not give in.

5. I love my silver/white, or shall we call it "Arctic blonde" coming in? The younger generation pay big bucks to have our natural grey/silver color, which is cool. I am so glad

I said *yes* to my natural sparkle. I wear my hair up a lot because when it is all back it looks as though I am fully silver.

6. My advice, listen to your inner nudge and know your why? My why was for my health. I didn't want the constant chemicals on my head. Lumps in my breast woke me up, and even though they turned out to be cysts, it still scared me. Enough was enough, I was going to do what it took to feel awesome from the inside out. I recommend you join a group to support you and help you through the tough days. Letting my sparkle come through aligns now with my top value which is *health*. What are your top values? Are you aligned with them?

Stories from the heart. They inspire. They encourage you. They make you believe that if they can do it, then you can do it. I am blessed that I have hundreds of stories in my Gorgeous Grey Movement Facebook group that I get to tap into daily for inspiration. These were just a few of the *brave* women who chose to share from their hearts in hopes of inspiring more women to own their sparkle. In the next chapter I will dive deeper into the topic of bravery. Our wish for you, my readers, is too *be brave* and join us in the sparkle movement.

CHAPTER EIGHT

My Super Heroes and My Brave Acts

"Transformation is the Journey you are on. You are exploring the wisdom of our soul. You are shedding old ways and beliefs that no longer fit who you are becoming. Be brave, dear one, you are becoming your authentic self."
—Author unknown

What does it mean to be brave? To take a chance? To risk it all? To color outside the box. To dare to be different. To break away from the pack. To learn to say *no* or *yes*. The word *brave* is defined as "having or showing mental or moral strength to face danger, fear, or difficulty: having or showing courage."[1] Where have you displayed bravery in your life? How did it feel before and after the event? Were you proud of yourself? Did it inspire you to continue to make more *brave* acts or pull back? Have you stopped being brave? Why did you stop? Or are you a brave one? What drives you to be brave? Did you have any heroes in your life to show you how to be brave? In this chapter I will share with you my brave heroes and how my stories of bravery have shaped who I am today.

Heroes. Hopefully you have had some heroes is your life. Who were they? When did you meet them? How did they help you move forward in your life? We all need heroes, wouldn't you agree? Some of you may call them mentors. They can shape who you are and who you want to become. They can be family members, friends, teachers, strangers, your boss, or a superhero you see in the movies or on TV. Let me introduce you to some of the people I have met along the way who became my heroes—and tell you what I learned from them.

My Dad

My dad was the most hard-working man I knew. He knew how to save his money for a rainy day and spend it on providing a good home for his family and putting food on the table. I learned about hustle and money from my dad. To this day I have always paid off my credit cards because he taught me to be smart with my money. "Don't spend money if you don't have it," he would say. He pushed us hard to hustle more and get another job to save to buy what we wanted. Yes, in grade 12 I had two jobs. I was a cashier at Safeway, which I loved, and I worked as a cashier at a gas station. Why two jobs? I needed to save for college (no free ride from my parents). I had a car that I paid for in cash and kept it running paying for gas, insurance, maintenance, and so on, and my dad charged me rent for my room. Let's be clear, I was upset that he charged me rent—$200 a month. I hadn't lived with my dad in years since my parents divorced, so this was a big change for all of us. I had already lived on my own since the age of seventeen, and I was scared to move back home. As a parent now, I totally understand why he did this. He wanted me to have a stake in my success. He didn't need my money, but he was teaching me another lesson: to be *responsible* for my success. This was his way of saying, "Hey, if you're serious about school this time, you need to grow up and show some financial responsibility as well." I needed those two jobs to be responsible for my *life*, and my dad wasn't giving me any handouts. To some that might seem harsh, but let me tell you, it taught me a lot about life and gave me the tools to land fast on my feet in the *real* world.

If you are a parent today, what lessons are you teaching your children about money and hustle? Are you having those tough conversations? Are you helping them become responsible adults? Do they know what hustle is? Do they save money and buy their own stuff? One of my favourite things to do with my girls is thrift shop. We love a good deal and finding treasures. Just a good wash, and they are good as new. Have you tried thrift shopping? It really is fun, and you save a ton of money. I once read an article about how to get rich; there were ten suggestions. Guess what one of them was, yep, you guessed it—thrift shopping.

Having two teens, I have taken the life lessons that were passed on to me and proudly passed them on to my girls. Both of them have had jobs since they were able to work. My ex and I are aligned with similar values on raising our girls, thank goodness! My heart goes out to all the single parents where that may not be the case. We have encouraged our daughters to save and buy their own phones and a lot of their extra clothes. They also have savings accounts that they cannot touch. Having clear expectations of what they each have to pay in their first year of university makes it easy for them to understand how much they need to save. We could hand them each $20,000 for their first year of post-secondary school since we have saved for four years of education for each of them, but what would that teach them? A free ride? Imagine each of them having to pay for their first year, do you think they would be better motivated to perform at a higher level? We think so! Thanks, Dad, for instilling the value of money and hustle in me; this has served me well.

My Mom

My mom is my Heart Hero. What did she teach me? How to love, help out in the community, and help people in need. After my parents' divorce when I was sixteen, we downgraded big time from a middle-class family to a lower-class family, not in *love*, but in finances. This is common, especially if the mother doesn't have the level of education and work experience to support a family. You see, my mom had me just after she turned eighteen and put her dreams on hold to be a mom to me, then my sister came along two years later, and then twelve years after that we said hello to my twin brothers. A single mom with four children and a grade II education unfortunately gets you minimum-wage jobs. She was hard working and would work several jobs to pay the bills. We struggled, but we got by. She even tried to run several network-marketing companies on the side to make an extra buck, but with very little success. Guess what, my mom never did get that pink Cadillac she was promised if she sold enough makeup. To say I was a little angry with all those companies promising money and a better life was an understatement. I remember coming home from school one day, and she was sold a $1,000+ vacuum cleaner that we didn't need with the hopes of using it as a demo to sell five in our area and earn it back for free. WTF! Well she never sold one vacuum cleaner.

Everyone in our neighbourhood was poor, at least I assumed they were. You see, we lived in what we called the "chicken coops," the cheapest townhouses in the area. Who would be able to afford one of those vacuum cleaners? Are you kidding me? (Note: this is the sixteen-year-old me speaking here, to give you an idea of the reaction I had back then around this topic of network marketing, aka NWM). Young teen *me* had another story that was forming big time: network-marketing companies are a scam, and people get hurt. Despite my strong opinion about NWM, the gift my mom gave me with NWM was the Tony Robbins cassette tapes she would make me listen to on our drives from Medicine Hat, Alberta, to Calgary. It was a three-hour drive to visit family. At first, I hated it and would just tune him out. Back then we didn't have sound-proof headsets, or I would certainly have bought a pair. But over time, Tony did find a special place in my heart, and I started to see the light of a better life.

Lucky for me and my sister, we were money hungry, so we started working as soon as we could to contribute to the household. Yes, we did use the food bank at times, and got gifts at Christmas from total strangers (thank you to the generous people when we needed you). I remember we also had photos from World Vision on our fridge because our mother made a monthly contribution to sponsor a few children in Africa, helping others even though we were so tight.

One of the jobs my mom had was as a lifeguard at the YMCA, and one day she met a foster boy named Todd, who was known to be a troublemaker. My mom got to know him

over the months and fell in love with his spunk. She consult-
ed my sister and me and asked us if she could foster Todd,
with the hope of adopting him down the road. Of course we
said *yes* and had an older brother living with us for a year.
Again, her heart was always bigger than her bank account,
but she still managed to pay the bills. She is still like this
today, always giving her money and time towards helping
others. Recently I saw a post from her travels in Ecuador,
where she was with her partner, Jim (best bonus dad in the
world), helping to build a home for a single mom with two
kids. Thank you, Mom, for showing me how to *love* others
and help those in need. I am forever grateful for your *gift*.

Yes, you guessed it, my "Love Language" is *words*, and my
mom figured that out long before the book came out. Thank
you, Mom. The book I'm referring to is *The 5 Love Languages:
The Secret to Love that Lasts* by Gary Chapman. It is a great
book that helps you discover your Love Language, as well as
your children's and your partner's. Knowing how I can show
them *love* and letting them know what's most important to
me has made a huge difference in my relationships. Just so you
know, gifts are my last love language, but send me a thank-you
card with sweet, truthful words, and you will melt my heart.

My Sister

My sister is my "everything hero." We had an interesting
childhood together, that is for sure. Most of our memories
are of moving around a lot, living in a broken family, or constantly fighting—more unhappy memories than good ones.
It's hard to believe that we made it through tough times and
came out as best friends. When did we start liking each other? you might ask. It was my second summer when I was

selling books door to door and I invited my sister to join me in the thirteen-week adventure across the country. She had witnessed the success of my first year and what I had been able to save, and she wanted some of that. So we ventured together in my red Toyota Corolla down to Tennessee for a week of intense sales training, and then up to the Peterborough area of Ontario, where we landed for the summer and would be roommates sharing the same bed. We hadn't lived together in years, so this was a big deal. We did cold-calling six days a week selling educational books and doing the grind so we could save money. That summer pulled us together. Listen, door-to-door sales is tough work. We had stories to tell every day of the jerks we would meet, but we also had beautiful stories of the kind people who took us in for a glass of water or food. There was something about sharing a "hard summer" together that brought us closer. My sister was my family, and we were there for each other to lean on when it was a good day or a bad day. It was just what we needed. From that summer on we were connected as soul sisters. We gained the love and respect for each other that has carried us through into our forties.

I moved to Ontario at twenty-five in 1995, and that was hard on everyone, especially my sister. I am still here in Ontario and she is in Calgary. We miss each other like crazy. The gift has been that she worked in the airline industry, which allowed for lots of travel (though never enough) to see each other, and that has helped keep our bond strong. We so cherish our time together, and we are always planning our next connection. Thank you, sister, for the amazing human being you are. You have taught me about love, friendship, loyalty, generosity, and always going the extra mile to keep our family connected. I am forever grateful for the bond that we have as sisters. We learned to forgive our past hurts and focused on rebuilding a beautiful forever relationship.

My Children, Ella and Sydney

My children are my playful heroes. My brave heroes. My forgiving heroes. My love heroes. Who would have thought that my children would be my greatest teachers about myself? The first thing my children taught me was how to play again, because, honestly, I had forgotten. With the daily tasks of adulthood, somewhere along the way I stopped playing. Everything seemed to be a task to be completed. I got caught in the grind of life: work, paying bills, doing chores, commuting, and repeat. I made very little time for fun. Have you ever been caught in the *grind* of life and forgotten about *play*? That was me until my children came along. They forced me to learn how to play again. Constantly they would be the ones pulling me away from my to-do list: "Come on, Mom, come play with us." It was always such an internal battle of "just wait" so I can finish the next thing and the next thing, only to have missed out on another opportunity for play. At times I would get irritated with them, only to find myself giving into the play request and putting the chore list on hold. It took me awhile to give myself permission to play and that play was just as important as the chore list. They really taught me how to play again. It was as if I had to relearn how to play like a kid. That was hard for me—anyone else? Why was it so hard for me to play like a child again? Was it because I felt I had grown up fast as a kid and went right into "adulting" that I just forgot how to play? Thank you, girls, for teaching your momma to slow down and learn how to play and have fun again in her child-like spirit. The funny thing about this journey is that now that they are teens and I am in a wonderful new relationship, I find myself playing more than they do and have to push them to come play more in the world.

Next came their brave acts. I got to witness many firsts. The first step, the first bike ride, the first bus ride, the first swim lesson, the first missing tooth, the first friend, the first fall, the first heartbreak, the first move, and their first family breakup of their parents. Many of these firsts had to happen with bravery in their hearts and cheerleading from the side by their family. I wonder if all kids are born with bravery in their hearts. They must to be able to move forward in life. I don't think you can move through life without brave acts. Their brave acts inspired me to look at where I needed to be *braver* in my life. As they get older, I have noticed that *fear* has crept in. Fear of speaking in front of the class. Fear of what their friends will think. Fear of going on that first date. Fear of learning how to drive. Fear of going on their first plane ride by themselves. When this happens, they need their parents to show them *bravery*. They need to hear from us where we were brave in our lives and how it turned out. I think it is important for our children to continue to see us being brave in our lives. Showing them that we don't stop being brave, but we keep pushing outside our comfort zones. I believe when we do this it gives them permission to be brave in their own lives. Thank you, girls, for your continued brave acts, as they keep me searching for more brave acts to accomplish in my own life.

Then came their Forgiveness. How many times have you said sorry to your kids? Sorry for yelling. Sorry for forgetting to pick them up at school because you were fast asleep on the couch. Sorry for not playing with them today. Sorry for breaking your promise to them again. Sorry for burning the grilled cheese again. Sorry for missing their practice. I realize I could write an entire chapter called "I Am Sorry, Kids." Oh my gosh! Anyone else? The best part of what I have learned from my kids is how fast they forgive. They know Mom is not perfect but that she is doing her best most days to be the best version of herself. I have good days and bad days, just like my kids. Together we learn how to say sorry and forgive quickly.

The last big lesson they have taught me was to love deeply. Nothing ever prepares you for the love of a child. The moment they are put in your arms for the first time. The tears of joys. The counting of the fingers and toes, knowing that they are healthy. The first sound. The first cry. The cutting of the cord. I think every parent can remember that first moment of *love* flooding their heart when they first meet their newborn. Despite the challenges that go with raising kids, and now teens for me, you keep coming back to that deep love connection that you have. Thank you, girls, for loving your momma hard!

Now it's your turn. Write down your list of heroes. What did they teach you? I dare you to send each of your heroes a card and thank them for the lessons they taught you.

- _____
- _____
- _____
- _____
- _____
- _____
- _____
- _____
- _____

- _____
- _____
- _____
- _____
- _____
- _____
- _____
- _____
- _____
- _____

Let's shift gears and talk about being brave. As defined on the first page of this chapter, the word *brave* means having or showing the strength to face danger, fear, or difficulty and having or showing courage. Would you not agree that going grey is a *brave* act? I think it is. Women say to me all the time, "Wow, you are so brave. I could never do that." I think that doing more *brave acts* in life gives you more strength to do more brave acts, such as going grey. Where do you need to step up and bring more bravery into your life?

Write a list of all the brave acts you can remember doing. Reflect on what you are most proud of. How you felt before you did them. How you felt afterwards. How old you were at the time.

- _____
- _____
- _____
- _____
- _____
- _____

- _____
- _____
- _____
- _____
- _____
- _____
- _____
- _____
- _____
- _____

Now write a list of the brave acts you are delaying doing in your life, and ask yourself why.

- _____
- _____
- _____
- _____
- _____
- _____
- _____
- _____
- _____
- _____
- _____
- _____
- _____
- _____
- _____
- _____

Here is a short list of my brave acts that I feel shaped who I am today:

- Moving to British Columbia from Alberta for a guy, whom I broke up with on my first day in BC because he cheated on me, but decided to stay there and finish my first year of university.
- Redoing grade 12 because I failed my first attempt
- Moving away from my family at age seventeen
- Giving up the opportunity to travel around the world with a best friend and deciding to take a corporate job
- Moving to Toronto by myself at age twenty-five to accept a job promotion
- Selling books door to door for two years without my dad's blessing
- Quitting my corporate job after ten years
- Going back to nutrition school for two years at age thirty-three
- Changing careers at age thirty-five
- Starting up a network-marketing company when I had little trust in them
- Speaking in front of five thousand people at conference
- Doing my first *live* broadcast on Facebook
- Leaving a twenty-year marriage
- Buying my first home by myself at age forty-five
- Writing a book
- Opening my heart again to *love*
- Running my first half-marathon

The cool thing about writing your own list is that you are reminded of all the brave acts that you have done in your life. How awesome is that! When I look at my list, I am proud and say to myself, "That wasn't so bad after all," even though in most cases at the time doing what I did was terrifying. I believe it was doing one brave act after another all these years that kept the momentum going, finally leading me to say *yes* to my sparkle. What one brave act can you do today that can start the momentum going in your life?

When I look back at some of the most terrifying decisions I had to make, most of the time they ended up taking me in a positive way to my next step in life. It was almost as if each decision was a test for my next step, and each next step shaped who I am today. I have a few stories I want to share with you that I feel impacted me the most.

Brave Act #1

Accepting a door-to-door job selling books while at university against my dad's wishes

This was a huge opportunity for me to spread my wings and move across the country, from Alberta to Ontario, and train in Nashville, Tennessee, for one week with some great sales training with world-class leaders. I did this job for two summers, 1992 and 1993. Thirteen weeks, six days a week, from 8 a.m. to 9 p.m. knocking on doors. Let me tell you, this work would shape me into the person I am today. I learned how to be persistent, work hard, sell, self-motivate during a rainy day, run my own successful business, get along with all types of people, and be open and teachable. It was some of the hardest work I ever had to do. I learned that people can be amazing and loving, opening their doors, feeding me dinner, offering me water or a dry place to stay. I also learned that people can be rude, judgemental, and can hurt you through words. In those two years I grew so much as a person and knew that if I could be successful doing this type of work, I would succeed at anything. Both years I landed in the top 5% of sales for North America out of four thousand students, not bad for a small-town girl from Alberta.

With the success came trips we could win. In my first year I won an all-paid trip to Hawaii, and the second year a trip to Mexico with my sister. That gave me the travel bug that I still have today. After my first year, I came home proudly with a $6,600 paycheque that I showed off to my dad because he had been so skeptical. It is amazing what we do to make our parents proud of us. To get their attention. I really wanted to prove my dad wrong, that I *could* do something like this and succeed. Of course, he was proud of me. I don't think he ever doubted I could not do it; as a parent, he was just fearful for my safety. Now that I'm a parent, I understand why he didn't want me to go as a young university student knocking on doors. As I mentioned before, the bonus in my second summer was rekindling my relationship with my sister.

This job experience stood out on my resumé no doubt. When I went to apply for all the jobs featured in the Business Commence Department at University of Calgary, my name was on most of the interview lists. I know it was this experience that got me in the door and eventually landed me a job in the food industry with a great company. Looking back, this experience set me up on a great career path. I was terrified of that job, but I knew deep down I needed to do something different and I did a brave act and it paid out.

Brave Act #2
Joining a network-marketing company
Let's loop back to the story about how I finally came to love network marketing (NWM). Remember my belief from childhood in NWM was low. When my mom introduced me to the concept of plant concentrates in a capsule fourteen

years ago, I said to her, "I eat well and I'm good." You see, I was already juicing, vita-mixing, cooking everything from scratch, and eating over ten+ servings of fruits and veggies. We also took a lot of expensive professional supplements. I thought we were rocking our health, and this was as good as it gets despite my crashing at 8 p.m. every night. I thought that having no energy was normal with a baby and a toddler. I also had a daughter who had a ton of allergies, so we lived in a bubble. After telling my mom no for many months, I finally caved. She called me after I'd spent two weeks with sick kids, and I was tired and vulnerable. I said yes. The yes was more to shut her up and prove her wrong. Why did I have to prove my mom wrong in my adult life? I secretly went behind her back and got a best friend to test Ella, Sydney, and me through live blood analysis before we added any plant concentrates. We went back four months later for testing, and my friend Anita was shocked that our health had improved so much, proven in our blood work. I told her how I had been feeling over the previous four months: more vitality, staying up longer, running again, and the kids had fewer sick days. I was starting to feel like me again. When you have kids back to back and breast feed for years, it really can deplete you, and that was me, a depleted momma bear. We took Ella for an allergy checkup and were shocked that her numbers had come down in half. I was so excited that we were finally starting to make some big steps forward in her health picture. Who would have thought that our family needed more plant matter to bridge the gap? But we did. We proved it in our blood that we were nutritionally deficient, and we had found a solution to top ourselves up. Anita was so impressed with our health improvements that she became my first distributor, and together we learned how to launch our NWM business. How cool to have a business with a best friend!

Fast forward a year and I ran my first half-marathon. Yeah me. This momma bear had her mojo back and we became an allergy-free family. Another wake-up call, we hadn't been eating enough plants, even though I thought we were. I got so excited about our health changes that I had to share with others. In my first year of sharing with friends and family I had over one hundred customers enjoying the added benefits of adding more plant concentrates to their diet. It was an easy button for clients, and even better, their kids were able to get it free on our Children's Health Study Program. But here's the thing, it was one of *those* companies. A network-marketing company that I had sworn I would never get involved in because of my story from childhood. Well let's just say it took four years for me to wear the T-shirt. I had the ITCS syndrome (I'm too cool syndrome). "I am a corporate gal, I am a nutritionist, this is beneath me" was my stinking-thinking. With enough education and stories of better health, I decided I could make this work. I saw average people creating above-average lives for themselves, and I wanted that. I wanted the *freedom* to say *yes*. To travel more. To play more. To raise my kids without childcare. As my marriage was crumbling, I had a choice to make. Plan to go back to my corporate career and be a slave to the boss, the commute, the grind, or decide to give it my all and partner with this on-line global-wellness franchise. Guess what I chose? My fear of never seeing my kids was enough to overcome my fear of NWM, and I went to work. I hustled (thanks to my dad I knew how to do that), and I built new relationships (thanks, Mom, for showing me how to love people), and I got out of my comfort zone over and over again. I learned how to become a network-marketing professional (thank you, Eric Worre, Dr. Mitra Ray, and Jeff Roberti, you rock). My NWM super-heroes.

I am happy to report that it worked. I love NWM. It allowed me to stay home and raise my kids on my terms. It allowed me to find me again, the Nicole I somehow lost along the way. It has given me the freedom of choice and adventure. What if I had let my fear own me? What if I never took this brave act? What if I had stayed in my comfort zone? I am forever grateful that my mom never listened to my no's. All she heard was "no, not right now." Today I have one of the largest organizations in Canada, impacting thousands of families with better health. I have become a top leader in our global company. I love working with women and watching them grow and make money to better their lives. I like to say, "I help women dream again." What a cool job that is? Who me, yes me! A small country girl from Medicine Hat, Alberta. I don't share this to brag but to let you know that anything is possible if you have a strong enough desire and hustle in your blood. Some of my best friends have come from my new global health tribe. A shout out to Melissa Hyde, whom I found on one of my business reports as an inactive rep. I was brave enough to call her one more time, and she picked up the phone this time. Divine timing for both of us. I invited her to an event and she said yes. That day changed our lives forever. She not only became my best friend, my travel partner, but also eventually a top producer in my organization. Why did this happen? Because I was brave enough to pick up the phone and ask her to an event. It is small brave acts that can change your life forever. Did you know that "Magic happens just outside your comfort zone"? This is a quote I have on my whiteboard, and it reminds me daily to play outside my comfort zone.

I am gifted with a freedom lifestyle that most people would only dream of. So, remember that sixteen-year-old girl who hated network marketing so much? Well look at her now, I couldn't imagine doing anything else. My point, my friends, is that if I can change a story from my childhood and turn it into a different story, then so can you.

What story do you need to change around your decision to go grey? Is that not the point of this book? Inspiring you to change your story just like I did to change my story on so many levels of my life. What wake-up call has been knocking at your door that you have been ignoring? What is your body saying to you? Are you listening to the whispers?

Brave Act #3
Leaving a twenty-year relationship

Never in a million years did I think I would go through a divorce. I had married for the forever partner. I didn't want to take the same path as my parents took. I remember the heartbreak from a child's perspective and didn't want my children to experience that same pain. When our marriage was unfolding and we were desperately trying to make it work, I remember thinking that it would be easier to commit suicide than to go through this pain. Crazy how the mind can play tricks. Crazy how the pain is so great that you so desperately think of an easier way. Yes, I thought about taking my own life. I remember exactly the night I wanted to leave this world. We were celebrating Christmas at my dad's house in Red Deer, and my husband and I had a big fight one night. I was so broken. I was so sad. I was so done on every level. I prayed that night for God to show me a sign that I needed to be here in this world because I believed the world would be better off without me. As I prayed and lay in the guestroom bed, my entire body started to glow and I saw lights flicker all around me. It was as if gold was painted all over my body and the room lit up. I started to cry and realized this was a divine sign telling me that I was needed. Even though we had spent a few years in counselling and were truly willing to save our marriage, I knew it was time to cut the cord. This was probably the most painful thing I have ever had to do, but in my soul I knew this was best for both of us. Our time together was up. We split as elegantly and respectfully as I could have asked for. No lawyers. No courts. Agreement to everything was done partly verbally and partly on paper. It took about a year to sell the house and set up two new homes, but we eventually made it happen. I am happy to report that we are both thriving in our lives. We do a great job co-parenting two amazing teens, and we are both in loving relationships. It is sometimes such a leap of faith when you decide to do a brave act, but when you do them often enough you just learn to *trust* and listen to your gut. Everything worked out better than expected. How cool is that! We are friends. We respect each other. We want the best for each other. Thank you, Arthur, for our twenty years together. We learned a lot. We grew. We made beautiful babies. We loved, but our time was up and we both knew it. I just had to be the one to pull the trigger. Hardest brave act I have ever had to do.

Brave Act #4
Loving again

Now as a single mom, I was trying to figure life out. I was taking a break from men and learning a new way of life. Splitting the kids 50% of the time was so hard for me. I cried myself to sleep for months feeling so much shame and guilt around my decision. I had to learn to live quietly on my own and re-invent myself again. Who am I? What do I love to do? What is best for my kids? How can I help them through this hardship? So much healing needed to happen. I eventually burned out my adrenals with the level of stress I was going through. It took me six months to bounce back and recover. What is adrenal stress? you ask. How do you know your adrenals are burned out? Most women I meet seem to have adrenal issues and need support.

Take the following adrenal stress test to see how your adrenals are doing. Write the number 1 beside the symptoms you have had in the past, 2 beside the symptoms that occur occasionally, 3 beside symptoms that occur often, and 4 beside symptoms that occur frequently, and then add up your score.

Adrenal Stress Indicator[2]	
Symptoms	Score
Blurred vision/spots in front of eyes	
Hormonal imbalances (i.e., thyroid problems)	
History of asthma/bronchitis	
Prolonged exposure to stress (i.e., job, family, caregiving)	
Headaches	
Environmental or chemical exposure or sensitivities	
Hypoglycemia/blood-sugar problems	
Food allergies	
Poor concentration/memory problems, mood swings	

Low energy, excessive fatigue	
Easily overwhelmed, inability to handle stress	
Post-exertion fatigue	
Dizziness upon standing (or fainting)	
Inflammatory conditions (arthritis, bursitis)	
Nervousness/anxiety, depression, irritability or anger	
Shortness of breath/yawning (air hunger)	
Cold hands or feet	
Low back pain, knee problems, sore muscles	
Insomnia/frequent waking	
Excessive urination	
Excessive perspiration or no perspiration	
Heart palpitations	
Edema of extremities or general edema	
Eyes light-sensitive	
Cravings: sugar, salt, coffee, or other stimulants	
Alcohol intolerance	
Recurrent colds or infections	
Digestive problems, ulcers	
Weight gain or weight loss	
High or low blood pressure	
Total Score	

If you scored ...

- Between 30 and 50: You've received an early-warning indicator that your adrenals are starting to weaken
- Between 50 and 80: Start with adrenal support
- Between 80 and 100: Your adrenals are taxed; you may want to take an adrenal glandular product

- Over 100: You are suffering from adrenal exhaustion and will require long-term adrenal support

My adrenal score was over 100. I knew I needed help. I always recommend getting professional help, such as from a naturopathic doctor, functional-medicine doctor, or holistic nutritionist, to support your healing. I used an ND to support my adrenals and get back on track. I still have to keep an eye on my symptoms because they can come back fast if I don't take care of myself. Sleep is my medicine now. I have given myself permission to gift my body with eight to nine hours of sleep each night because that is what I seem to need to thrive. The old Nicole would brag about getting five to six hours of sleep so I could get everything done in a day. Now I just prioritize and make sure my A list gets done, and the rest can wait until tomorrow. I value health too much now to worry about the to-do list.

Back to learning to love again. After I had healed my body from adrenal fatigue and started to feel good again about me, I started to online date. I think this is an important point, ladies: Heal your body, mind, and spirit *first* before you go hunting for your next partner, or you'll be at risk of attracting the same old energy that will not serve you well. Online dating—OMG! I could write an entire book about this chapter in my life. The crazies, the liars, the fakes, and the users. After a year-and-a-half of dating some decent men and some not-so-decent men, I decided to take another break. A clearing was needed. I seemed to be attracting the same unhealthy male energy. After a well-needed break and more spiritual healing, I was clear about what I was looking for. I created a list of over one hundred qualities I was looking for in a mate, as well as one hundred qualities I felt I could offer. I wrote the list in my beautiful journal, and I would read it daily along with this poem:

Dear God, I am ready to accept into my life a loving partner who will complement my own energy, who will provide open and honest communication, who will assist me as I assist him in experiencing life, with the intention of allowing our souls to grow to their fullest potential. God, I ask that you help me in opening my heart to feel this person. Love and guide us together. Amen

After a few months of this work and clarity, we finally met online. It started off as friendship—passionate dates and great conversations about life. I wasn't jumping into anything serious and neither was he. We took our time. Our souls connected. We fell in love. He gave me hope again that *love* was possible. He slowly brought my walls down and showed me what Love could feel like again. We act like kids playing together in this amazing world. We have so much in common and we accept each other for who we are. This is the first relationship I have ever had where I feel no judgement. He accepts me for me. Talk about *freedom*. Maybe because I stopped judging myself and allowing others to take my power away. Thank you, Bradley, for coming into my life and teaching me patience and how to *love* again.

Brave Act #5

Going silver at age forty-seven—OMG!

When I finally decided that I was going to let my grey hair come in, I had so many fears and doubts. Now that I am ten months in, there is no turning back. I am in. No questions.

No doubts. This is my forever hair. This is me. But go back a year and I would have called you crazy. No way; I would never do that. I am too young. I am in a new relationship and need to look *good*. I am a health professional; there is an image I have to live up to. Wow! The stories we create in our heads. My only regret is not doing it when I was thirty-five, but I guess I wasn't ready then. The new Nicole is ready for this amazing transformation. I now realize that all my stories and brave acts have led me here. I now get to be a "sparkle hero" for someone else. It's my time to step up with this brave act because I am ready. I am ready to be that *sparkle hero* that women are looking for. Here I am.

As I close this chapter, I want to let you know that this was an emotional chapter for me to write. I had many tears and doubts about how vulnerable I could be with you. It was a chapter that I needed to share to help heal my past. I let my heart do the talking, and I know that there are messages in here for everyone to benefit from. My message to you is take on a brave act that you have been avoiding and become your *own hero* of your life.

CHAPTER NINE

We Are Not Alone

"Our life's path is revealed to us by spiritual guideposts. They mark the way and lead us to our soul's ultimate purpose."

—RANDI G. FINE

I didn't make the decision to go grey overnight, as you have figured out by now. Since my early thirties, it has been a deep dive into personal growth. Finding out who I am. What I like? What I stand for? What my values are? What I want in life? Lots of healing; lots of forgiveness; lots of letting go. And lots of spiritual awakenings and nudges that have led me to this Sparkle transformation. Along the way I was gifted with amazing spiritual mentors who have shown up in my life to help me on this path of self-awareness and self-love. In this chapter I share with you how my spiritual path unfolded and introduce you to the spiritual heroes who impacted me the most.

I was introduced to God as a child through my mom. She took us to a number of different churches, where we learned Bible teachings. My first Bible was a Christmas gift from my grandma Havel when I was eight. After my mom's divorce, we seemed to stop going to church as she was learning to find her way again in life. I too slowly lost my way to my connection to God. I stopped praying and probably even stopped believing. It wasn't until I had my girls that I started thinking about my spiritual connection and what I would teach my girls. I shopped around for a year to find the right church for our family. The most suitable one I finally found was in Toronto, which meant a commute of over an hour, and this wasn't going to work for our family with young kids. The idea of attending church as a family fizzled out and I dropped the search. Then a special encounter with a friend of mine, Adriana, planted a seed and got me thinking about "divine energy."

Adriana Girdler and I met in 1995 through work. I remember our first sales meeting at an Italian restaurant in Etobicoke. We were both sales reps for Cadbury Beverages; she had the Windsor territory and I had the Greater Toronto area. We instantly connected and we became long-distant friends. She eventually moved on to other work and moved away, and we lost touch. This was before social media, so losing touch with people was quite common. Then a beautiful connection happened. One evening in Burlington, Ontario, a colleague of mine ran into Adriana at an oyster bar, and she told her that I lived in the area. She gave Adriana my phone number and we reconnected after years apart. Guess what, she also lived blocks away from me—OMG! We picked up exactly where we had left off. We spent lots of time together. We celebrated with each other over our first pregnancies and first big promotions. She even inspired me to resume running, even in the winter at 6 a.m. She was hard core, me—not so much, but I didn't want to let her down so I would often drag my lazy butt out to run with her. After three years together, I moved cities away and we saw less and less of each other. Finally, months had gone by and we had arranged a friendship date at a mall halfway between us. Something big happened at that lunch: Adriana stopped talking and looked me straight in the eyes as tears started running down her face. She asked me, "Do you see it Nicole?"

"See what" I asked.

"The white light that is connecting both our hearts. It is so beautiful. I have never seen anything like it," she said. I couldn't see this light, but I knew she had seen it. It touched her big time, and she was taken aback. At that moment the seed for the idea that an energy outside of us was planted, and that you could actually see it. I was fascinated, but Adriana was even more fascinated.

Next stop was a book store. She wanted to learn about what had just happened and why. Why could she see the light and I couldn't? Was it just in her head or did she really see it? That started her on her path to a spiritual awakening, and I was right behind her—I just didn't know it. I was much slower on my path, but I got to witness from a distance the transformation that was taking place in my friend. It was beautiful. She found a spiritual coach and started her journey to understanding divine energy. Since that day, Adriana has incorporated spirituality into her life and business practices, using it to guide her (see the resources section on page 235). I am so proud of Adriana for her self-awareness and how she touches many lives with her spiritual gifts. A seed was planted in our hearts that day over lunch. Divine is wonderful.

My next encounter with a mentor would happen at a library in Richmond Hill, Ontario. When I was studying holistic nutrition at the Canadian School of Natural Nutrition, we had to take a course on mind, body, and spirituality. It was my favourite class. It lit me up. I was listening to my body. I wanted to dive back into what this meant for me. Around the same time, my nutrition networking group was hosting a special guest speaker at the library on spirituality. I signed up and was excited to learn. That special guest, Caroline Dupont, became one of my heroes who would set my spiritual path on fire. She grabbed my attention with her own personal journey and talked about the idea of a spiritual practice using energy modalities such a reiki. Her story of how she discovered the spiritual world made me curious, so I booked an appointment. I remember going to her home, where I was led to a small room with a massage table and chair. Her partner at the time was lying on the table, and Caroline was going to channel spirit guides as she performed reiki on him. I thought this was crazy, but I was willing to go along with it. As we got deeper into the session, she asked me to start asking questions. Messages were coming through him from the divine and being channelled into the room. I had never experienced this before. Spirit was speaking through him to me. I had asked questions that neither of them would know about me personally, and Spirit was bang on. I was in shock and disbelief that this divine energy was actually an entity. The session took about two hours, and it left me feeling excited but also still very confused. To have your first divine encounter with spirit energy was scary, but it also gave me hope.

As I mentioned, I was raised in the church. My mom bounced us around from church to church looking for answers. After a while, I was a disillusioned child of God, not really believing, and in my teens and twenties I stopped believing. To come back to the possibility that we are all connected to divine energy and that God energy is in us was like going back full circle. That appointment was a catalyst for me to begin my own spiritual growth, so thank you, Caroline, for the gift you shared with me that day in your home. I am forever grateful. She was my first spiritual hero—a seed was planted and I started to water it.

My next mentor came through a referral from a colleague to her friend Jade, who did spiritual work using Ayurvedic principles. I called and booked my first appointment with Jade in her home. Who would have known that Jade would be my next spiritual hero? I spent a few years with her learning and connecting through her beautiful teachings. As an Ayurvedic practitioner, she taught me so much about the Indian practice of foods, oils, massage, and connection that helped me become a better nutritionist. I was a case study for her for an Ayurvedic massage, and one day she had made a special dough for me and brought it from her kitchen to the treatment room. As I lay on the table, she wrapped the dough in a circle around my heart. Then she filled the circle of dough with custom-made oils and let the oil settle into my heart chakra as she worked on the rest of my body. I had never experienced anything like this. There was so much peace and love in my heart that I started to cry. Could I feel this type of self-love for myself more often? Could I love more deeply with my family? Could I feel this type of peace when I left this room? All I know is that I felt so amazing and I wanted to feel more of this.

Jade had finally helped me discover a new way of feeling. She taught me about self-love and how that could feel. Little did I know that this would be my last session with her as she soon passed away from cancer. In all our treatments together, she never once mentioned that she was sick. I noticed a few things, such as that her hair was cut short, allowing her natural grey to show. She said her grey was a positive step in staying healthy in her quest for being a better holistic practitioner. I thought she was so brave. She always brought her best game to our sessions and always focused on my healing. She was such a selfless woman in a time when she was fighting for her life. Jade, I wish I had a chance to thank you for the work we did together. You left this physical world much too soon, but you impacted so many lives through your *love* and your *gifts*. You helped me in so many ways, and you became a spiritual hero for me in my early days of finding myself again. Thank you, Jade, for our short time together. You are an angel of *love*. My spiritual hero.

In 2008 Jade introduced me to my next spiritual mentor, Joy. When our family moved to Uxbridge, Ontario, into our new home, I felt other energies in the house. Some might call them ghosts or entities. Whatever they were, we didn't feel welcome. Joy's practice was diverse in the spiritual world. One of her gifts was being able to communicate with the spiritual world, and even see spirits. Was I skeptical about this type of work? Yes! Why? Because I had never experienced it before and had only heard stories of people with this skill. I was as skeptical as anyone, but I trusted Jade. Joy fit my family in within a day from when I had called her. She lived nearby, and when she arrived at our home, she walked the property and then explained to me that we did have spirits, which she called entities, that didn't want us there and were causing trouble. This would explain all the fighting and heavy energy we experienced during the first week we lived in our dream home. Once Joy "cleared" the house and property, we instantly felt the shift in energy. It was incredible! I became a believer in this work. Another spiritual hero showing up in my life and showing me another element of this spiritual world.

Shortly after we moved into our country property, my youngest daughter, Sydney, became very sick. She was always congested and seemed to have a constant cold that she couldn't get rid of. This was my healthy child, so to have her go downhill go quickly made me very concerned. The rest of the family didn't get colds, but we were struggling with fatigue. I asked around town who the "go-to" holistic professional would be, and Jennifer Hough's name came up many times. I looked her up and learned that she had the largest holistic-nutrition practice in Canada. Wow, impressive, and right in my community. I booked an appointment with her a few weeks out and drove up to her place in the country. Within ten minutes she picked up the culprit: Mold. How did she know this so quickly? Because she was dealing with the same problem in her own home, and she had similar symptoms to Sydney. OMG! Is that not *divine* intervention guiding me to the perfect person to help us? She gave us some remedies and some volcanic rock packages to place all over the basement to help pull out toxins until we had it properly assessed. Sure enough, we had mold all over the basement and had to do an immediate renovation to the basement as well as replace our furnace. Once we did all the renovations and removed the mold and detoxed our bodies with special supplements, Sydney's health returned and the rest of the family's energy bounced back. Black mold is very dangerous and is considered to be a slow poison that damages people's health.

After Sydney was healed from mold exposure, I continued to book appointments with Jennifer for my own health and for her mentorship. She was a holistic nutritionist, but she had also been incorporating spiritual coaching, workshops, and healing sessions that intrigued me. I was at a crossroads in my life regarding what to do for a career. I had just shut down my nutrition practice in Maple and moved to a new area. I was casually doing my NWM business, but I still had the "I-am-too-cool-for-NWM syndrome," so I was hesitant about going out to share in my new community. I didn't want to be known as the NWM gal. Remember, my resistance to NWM had been at a very deep level from childhood. I still had the charge of a sixteen-year-old, and I obviously hadn't yet healed that part of me. Jennifer had offered me the opportunity to sign up for her one-year mentorship program, but money was tight. I knew deep down that I needed this, so I said yes and trusted I would figure out how I would pay for it.

During the first six months of working with her, I had ventured off and created a new company, "Passion for Nutrition." I would go back to the food industry that I knew so well, leverage all my contacts, and consult on cleaning up the food labels. I was going to save people from all those toxic ingredients and help them make healthier choices. They were going to love me. Well, after six months of banging my head against a brick wall, I started to realize that the food industry wasn't ready for me. They weren't willing to change. I was so deflated; what was I going to do? Should I start a nutrition practice all over again, which would include evenings and weekends and missing out on family time? That didn't feel right either. I remember Jennifer each month asking me, "Are you listening to the nudges the universe gives you daily?" I know I was resisting for sure, and she knew it too. She wanted me to get quiet before I started each day and just listen. She wanted me to meditate. Some days I would, and other days I would not. I resisted this practice big time, yet she kept telling me that it works and to trust. As I started asking for more help from the universe to show me the next step, guess what signs the universe kept showing me. More orders were coming in from my NWM business, and more distributors were calling me to start working again. Are you kidding me? Seriously, Universe, you want me to do NWM? Jennifer really helped me through this crossroads in my life—the battle between ego and heart. After one year of working with her, I was strong enough to say yes to my NWM business and start wearing the T-shirt proudly. Who would have thought that my investment with Jennifer would lead me to becoming one of the largest NWM teams in Canada? Do you see how the divine is so good if you listen? Have you been resisting the nudges? The whispers? Isn't it time you started to listen? The universe tries to get you back to your soul purpose. The path I was put on has been incredible and has filled my soul. It is *a knowing* that this is where I need to be. I am a leader. I am a mentor. I am a health coach. I am me. I am free. Thank you, Jennifer, for the gifts you have shared with me to allow me to open my heart and trust my nudges. You are my spiritual hero.

Over the years I was introduced to or shown other wonderful spiritual mentors who continued to share their knowledge and deep understanding of the divine energy and how to work with it. I learned to ask for help and guidance; you might call it prayer or meditation practice. I remember once having a challenging morning with one of my daughters; divorce was still fresh for our family, so we had some very emotional days, and this was one of them. After I got my daughters off to school, I needed to go clothes shopping to get ready for a big conference I was attending in California. Before I went out into the world, I asked for help. Please, God, send me someone who can help our broken family heal from the divorce. Let me tell you, the universe can work fast if you are ready. That morning at Winners in Stouffville, about twenty-five minutes away from home, who would have thought that I would meet my next spiritual healer in the shoe section? She came flying around the corner asking me what I thought of her shoes, and I was immediately drawn to her energy. We chatted, I got the same shoes as she did, and we both knew we were meant to meet. When we exchanged business cards, we were both amazed. She had been guided that morning to go shoe shopping, and I had been guided to head to that store, which I only had been to only a few times. She looked at me and said, "You sell plant concentrates in a capsule."

"Yep, that's me, the veggie crack lady." What I learned later was that she was a cancer survivor and she hated eating fruits and veggies. To her, I had been an angel in helping her build back her strong body and offering the "easy button" she had been looking for. I looked at her card and said, "You're a spiritual healer."

"Yep," she said, and I thought that maybe she was the one who could help my family heal. Well, she was. I worked with Zak for a few years. She not only helped my girls but also took my healing from the past to a whole new level. I did some of the deepest emotional work with her that I had ever done before. It was crazy what I had buried from my past. One traumatic event that I had buried so deeply was that I had been raped at the age of sixteen at a party, and I never told anyone because I felt so ashamed and embarrassed. This pain closed off my root chakra, preventing me from fully experiencing my true feminine self. It was after about six months of working with Zak on the afternoon of a full moon when we both felt the pain energy leave my body. We cried together. I finally gave my body permission to release this old stuck energy that was holding me back on so many levels. My root chakra was finally open, and I was ready to experience a new way of being. Another level of self-love was unfolding. Where in your life do you need to heal past wounds to move forward? Are you willing to dig deep and go to the dark place? I know it is scary, but it will be so worth it. I trusted Zak to do this deep work with me. She also became a business colleague and a dear friend. The universe answers if you ask. Thank you, Zak, my spiritual hero.

My next mentor was Jenny. She was introduced to me by my business mentor, Dr. Mitra Ray. Jenny and I worked together for months, helping me to hit an important milestone in my business while getting certified for Reiki Level One. That was an amazing experience, not only for hitting my business goals but also for learning how to work with energies myself. Thank you, Jenny, my Spiritual Hero.

Last summer a colleague and I jumped on the phone to catch up, and she happened to mention her spiritual coach. She thought for sure I would have heard of Winnie, but I hadn't. Again, I became curious and had to book a session with her. Winnie is a beautiful soul who helped me expand to the next level. We hit it off and we have been working together since last September. The first time I walked into her healing room, she cautioned me about the energies in the room. I didn't really know what to expect. I could feel the energy. The room went from cold to hot in an instant. It felt as though my skin was being tickled and an energy surrounded me, making me feel supported and safe. I knew this is where I needed to be. It was a knowing. I was at peace.

After our first session on a Friday, the next morning at 4 a.m. I felt Spirit wake me up. I decided to mediate, and I felt the divine energy and messages pour into me. I began writing while in this meditative state. When I came out of the meditation, I didn't even remember what I had written, and the rest is history. What an experience to be able to listen to the divine messages! The first time I heard that this was even possible was from Wayne Dyer. I loved his teachings. He told his readers that this was often how he would write. I remember thinking, "How cool to be so spiritually connected that you trust yourself enough to share a message with the world." Well, it really happened to me to. I guess I had done enough spiritual work—for about fifteen years—before I was connected enough to trust and listen. Thank you, Winnie, for the deep spiritual work we did together. You are a gift. You are a spiritual hero.

So now you have had a peek into my world of spiritual heroes who have shown up at the right time, each teaching me something new and helping me expand into the person I am today. Every one of my teachers played a special part in my journey. I don't think I would have decided to "own my sparkle" so soon had I not done the spiritual work first. When I was asking to find the right publishing company, I got enough signs to call Dawn James and connect with her. I instantly knew that she would be the perfect fit for my book. We knew each other from years earlier in a women's networking group, and social media kept us in touch. Later I would realize that she is also a spiritual hero to many people around the world, and I am fortunate to have her as my spiritual book coach. How awesome is that! Thank you so much, Dawn, for keeping me on my path to launching this book when in the beginning I didn't believe in myself as a writer. My closing message for you if you feel lost and are searching for a clearer path is to consider learning how to connect to the divine energy daily and listen to the whispers. Maybe your next spiritual hero is waiting for you just as they were waiting for me. You are not alone!

Finally, I thank you, dear readers, for providing a safe place for me to share my vulnerability, my story, my pain, my fear, my heart, and my passion. I hope that my acts of bravery will inspire you to have the courage to perform brave acts. Thank you to all the brave grey heroes who have gone before us to inspire this Sparkle Movement! If you aren't ready yet to go grey, that is okay. I don't judge you. I have offered you a lot of heathier options so you can do it in a healthier way for you and for the environment. For those who are ready to embrace the grey, welcome to the Sparkle Movement and enjoy your new-found freedom. I will end with a favourite quote from Theodore Roosevelt:

> It is not the critic who counts; not the man who points out how the strong man stumbles, or where the doer of deeds could have done them better. The credit belongs to the man who is actually in the arena, whose face is marred by dust and sweat and blood; who strives valiantly; who errs, who comes short again and again, because there is no effort without error and shortcoming; but who does actually strive to do the deeds; who knows great enthusiasms, the great devotions; who spends himself in a worthy cause; who at the best knows in the end the triumph of high achievement, and who at the worst, if he fails, at least fails while daring greatly, so that his place shall never be with those cold and timid souls who neither know victory nor defeat.

Big sparkle hugs,
Nicole Scott

APPENDIX

Following are stories some of my spiritual coaches have written as messages to you.

Caroline Marie Dupont
Soul Coach, Meditation and Yoga Teacher, Holistic Nutritionist

Greetings, dear readers,

First, I want to remind you that as you hold this book in your hands, you are already exactly where you need to be on your journey. Although I will be sharing some threads of my life as I continue to awaken to my true self, your unfolding is precious in its uniqueness as it reflects your soul's gifts and plans for this lifetime.

Although I have some recollection of being interested in living from my highest self at a very early age, like most of us, many of those inner soul nudges got hidden behind efforts to fit in at home and at school during my teen years.

It wasn't until the birth of my first child in my late twenties, after having married my professional hockey player husband and obtained a master's degree in exercise physiology that I began to feel a strong desire to live from a more authentic place. Meeting my children ignited my heart. They were shockingly fresh and soulful! Through them I became painfully aware of my conditioning and was naturally very curious about how to let that go. The awakening and accelerated soul growth at that time began to thaw out my emotional being, which had become rigidified behind a façade of efficiency and "perfection." This was very challenging for me because up until then I hadn't developed the skills and perspectives to relate in a healthy way to my emotions.

Of course, like you, as my inner world was shifting, I was drawn to many new interests that would contribute to my healing and also inform my vocation as a holistic health practitioner. For example, holistic nutrition, particularly plant-based eating, became a strong passion that continues to this day. The changes in food choices amplified the spiritual shifts that were affecting every part of my life. I was compelled to share what I was discovering through cooking classes, teaching for the Canadian School of Natural Nutrition, and eventually writing several health, nutrition, and recipe books.

I became disillusioned with mainstream fitness, where I had been a personal trainer and fitness-class leader, choosing to let that go and instead to train for and lead Nia classes (a holistic movement form that blends dance, yoga, martial arts, and therapeutic movement). Later I would certify as a yoga instructor and currently love teaching restorative yoga in particular because of its meditative pace with opportunities to inhabit the body, welcome emotions, establish a healthy relationship with the mind, and touch into Presence.

When I came across the concept of energy in the early days of my awakening, it resonated deeply and helped me to make sense of my world. I studied several forms of energy work and began practising on clients. Later it felt enlivening to work with energy intuitively, and I continue to find that having an ongoing relationship with it enriches my daily life and my work as a soul coach and teacher.

Slowly but surely my personal tool box was expanding as I simply followed my interests and paid attention to what life was putting in front of me. Looking back, I can see that there was never a time when life wasn't providing for me. It was natural to share those modalities that I had aligned with and also to give myself the freedom to intuitively adapt them to my needs and those of my clients.

It felt exhilarating to wake up to a perspective of myself and of life that felt deeply grounding and simultaneously expansive and full of possibilities. At the same time, and perhaps paradoxically, I continued to be painfully aware of the emotions that I had been carrying, and of the unhealthy patterns that ran through just about every aspect of my life. The early years of my conscious spiritual journey were extremely challenging. They included frequent moves as our financial situation deteriorated, my marriage ending, and feeling a great deal of stress in just about every aspect of my life.

With much support, seen and unseen, I managed to rebuild my life as a single mother of two children, business owner, and householder. My unwavering priority through it all has been to cultivate a direct relationship with my soul. I've always had a deep interest in the possibility of waking up to my true nature in the midst of mainstream life, and to be of service. I sensed that this would ultimately be the most direct way to create my beautiful life. I believe that many of us are taking on this challenge nowadays. Whereas in the past those of us who were spiritually inclined would have secluded ourselves in monasteries and ashrams, in this lifetime we are ready to experience the richness of living a spiritual life in the midst of regular life with responsibilities, jobs, partners, children, and so on.

For me, although much of life was simply meeting each ordinary moment with the highest version of myself that I could access, I also had some extraordinary mystical experiences that expanded my view of reality and my curiosity around what life was really about. I believe that once we touch into a longing for spiritual connection, we all begin to have contact with the mystical side of life in ways that speak to our uniqueness.

For example, in 2004 a series of events led to a fortuitous meeting with a man who discovered a profound gift for channelling while receiving energy work from me. As his gift unfolded, we were guided to offer readings to private clients and occasionally large groups. Over the course of the next two years, I was in ongoing direct contact with my spirit guides (including Edgar Cayce) through him and received an education on the path of the soul, particularly how it relates directly to our well-being: how to connect to our true nature and how our challenges, health, and otherwise are simply and always a form of guidance from a benevolent God/Creator/Universe.

The time spent with my guides deepened my commitment to exploring my reality through meditation. In addition to a regular practice, I began to attend silent retreats, particularly with the American spiritual teacher Adyashanti, but also with people in his lineage, including his wife, Mukti, and Sharon Landrith. Having attended and led many silent retreats, I've consistently found that conditioning simply dissolves in the radiant light of presence that arises in the midst of prolonged silence and stillness, revealing an ever more natural and evolved version of ourselves.

In my work today I'm most interested in guiding people to recognize their inherent wholeness regardless of current circumstances. We are not broken and we don't need to be fixed. Our conditioning and patterns, although distorted, were all innocent attempts to survive and fit into a world that doesn't honour the soul. As we awaken to a sincere desire to live from the radiance of our true natures, and when we aren't fighting what is, our energy gets freed up to align with Life and our soul's unique unfolding within it.

Dear reader, live your own story. Take responsibility. Ask for help. Be as you are. And, enjoy yourself!

Love,

Caroline

Zak Lioutas
Spiritual Elder, Master Key Holder, Soul Activator, Meditation Teacher

We don't always know why things have happened for us the way they have happened, but we learn to accept it and move on knowing that we have learned the lessons of the past and are willing to create change in our future.

The past doesn't define who we are, it creates this character of who we want to become, leaving behind suffering, trauma, and beliefs that were embedded within our souls. Taking on the wisdom and guidance to understand that there is something greater for us out there. Something that ignites the spark within us. Something that brings us greater pleasure in knowing, that what we are seeking is also seeking us.

The Universe works in mysterious ways. Regardless of what journey we have crossed, we must sing psalms of forgiveness and gratitude.

Life hasn't always been this simple and the above hasn't always been this easy to understand or deal with. When you learn to climb the ladder out of darkness, you learn that in life there's more of what we want or don't want that will come towards us.

It's literally up to our own minds, actions, and reactions to what comes before us and what we want to create or what we walk away from.

Happiness is a choice we need to make, it's not our children's, spouse's, friends', or co-workers' responsibility to make us happy. We are responsible for our own happiness and creating it the way we want it to be. Remembering that others can only amplify our happiness, and if they don't we have the power to walk away from what doesn't make us happy or feel good.

Spiritual awakening happens when we get in our own way and think we can do everything on our own, leaving ourselves depleted, resentful, angry, and confused with what life is trying to tell us.

Layers of healing and working though the ego are the most challenging tasks any human can take on, especially when things don't make sense or work out the way we believe they should.

We must dance with fear, self-doubt, guilt, anger, and resentment to find the seed within our own beings that lights us up and makes life feel orgasmic and free. Getting naked in our truth unapologetically and poetically, not needing anymore validation from the outside world, starts to empower us. The sensation of faith becomes stronger, trusting becomes inevitable.

At the age of three I saw my first spirit. It wasn't easy living in this world of duality, which wasn't spoken about or accepted as it is today. I had to hide from being authentically me, leaving me feeling depressed and disconnected from my own purpose in life, as I was pleasing others around me and bringing comfort to their needs, rather than bringing comfort to my own self.

In my teens, until cancer struck in my twenties, drugs, sex, and booze were my escape to fill in an empty void that was temporary relief with long-term effects of emotional suffering and trauma. Drugs, whether a substance or an emotion, are drugs.

When we look at the intention of why we react a certain way, we recognize that we are filling a void of attention we may be seeking to belong to or to disconnect from.

What we feed energy to, feeds us in return. Whatever void we are trying to fill in another's truth is the absence to our own truth, and power. I can tell you first hand that owning your power and standing in your truth isn't always easy. I can also tell you that it's extremely orgasmic and liberating when you open yourself up and speak your truth in a compassionate way and start receiving the Universe's pleasures, then life takes a whole new trajectory.

Spirituality is about living every day in the comfort of being naked in your own skin of truth and truly loving yourself and humanity in a way that makes your body quiver and your divine juices drip.

We must not deny our sexual needs. Our divine soulful juice sprinkled in Gaia is the greatest gift we can give ourselves. Opening yourself up isn't only about giving unconditionally, it's also about receiving unconditionally in all areas of your life, physically, financially, and sexually. Are you ready to live in your truth and stand in your power in a bold, fierce, unstoppable way?

My purpose is to empower women to manifest the lives they are destined to live by dissolving mental and emotional challenges and activating their souls. As I share my lenses in guiding women to live their best lives, it naturally arouses their yonis (wombs) to beat to their hearts' drums.

Learning to trust the process and let go of the past, becoming present in the now and future, and creating healthy boundaries in all areas of your life by making yourself the priority allows you to serve another in your fullness.

The greatest advice I can give anyone is to find someone you align with and start working with them if you are ready to take a leap with life and its pleasures. You will save yourself a lot of pain, suffering, time, and money when you have someone who can see your light and can guide you, rather than trying to figure it out on your own.

Know that you are worth the investment in healing your soul. You are not alone, the Universe is always watching and guiding you, the choice is yours of what path you want to take.

Zak

Wineke (Winnie) Engelage
Owner/Operator at Core Soul (core-soul.com/ winnie)

First of all, I AM so excited for Nicole. I know her book, full of wisdom and inspiration, will serve so many women on this planet. I feel very blessed to be part of Nicole's life in some small way.

How fitting is this chapter? We are not alone! We can feel so alone and different while journeying through parts of our lives. We can let titles and labels define us, and that can make us feel even more alone as we are not being our authentic selves. This is where I come in. I am known as a "quantum shift facilitator" and "New Earth Transformational guide." What does that even mean? you ask. Quantum Healing is a powerful energetic form of healing and shifting that takes place in the Quantum Field. The healing that I do occurs on the level of the DNA—a level that is much deeper than many other types of energetic healing. It can be done in person or long-distance.

I AM thankful that I get to share a few pieces from my journey with the hope that these droplets of insight will assist your Soul and Path upon this Earth.

I AM fully embracing this new Earth experience. I have been groomed since birth by beautiful guides and beings of light so I can be part of the awakening of the Souls on the Planet. What a rewarding and humbling experience this is! I have so much Gratitude for all that is unfolding and for all the Souls that step up to the plate and make a difference for themselves and others. We are affecting the collective Consciousness, Humanity, The Earth, and beyond. How magical is that! My guides and I are here to remind *you* that we are all paying it forward when we give ourselves the gift of self-work. We are here to share the energy of our Infinite Soul and the Light of our own personal truth. Remember to have trust and faith. I believe we were all born with a purpose, but sometimes we forget that purpose or just plain ignore it. My work involves helping people connect back to that Soul purpose. My Soul orchestrated monumental challenges for me to get back into my Soul purpose.

The "messages" and "nudges" became louder and louder in my mid-forties. I had gotten away from what I was called to do here on the Planet. Looking back at it all, I must say that the Universe and my team of guides have an excellent sense of humour, if I may say so myself. At times they had to bring me back kicking and screaming. I became very sick in order to align and shift back into my authentic Soul purpose. They gave me two options. Shift (heal) myself and do what I agreed to do on the Planet or waste my gifts and health. It was shared that there would be no coming back from the next round. I knew on all levels that my stroke was here to show me the fearful and dark place I was in. I had allowed myself to give the most precious parts of my Soul and joy away to fear and anxiety. The pain bodies that needed attention, became louder and louder. In addition to the stroke, I had to make amends with the pain of not ever having my own children. A full hysterectomy was decided after a tumour was detected. That indicated I had to heal my Divine Feminine and Ancestral lines as well. Then rheumatoid arthritis with painful bone spurs coming out of my feet and hands was thrown in for good measure as well. It became overwhelmingly clear and obvious I had ignored almost every sign that my body brought to me. In the end. Rock bottom is where I started.

With all my health scares, I was ready to listen to the screams of my body. I handed in my resignation at my job and started my healing journey. I had to revisit deep core issues. I worked through childhood traumas, fears, loss, death, and abandonment. As well, many other pain bodies resurfaced that I had to heal. Then I had to learn Forgiveness, which has been a big part of my personal healing journey.

In addition to my healing, I embraced meditation, qi gong, and yoga. I followed my inner guidance and was brought to facilitators all over the world. Feelings of unworthiness melted away. Clarity appeared. I also became certified in

Energy Medicine and Energy Psychology. Once I made the decision to be free again, the right teachers and opportunities came my way. My decision to do the self-work set me free. I AM happy to report I successfully healed every aspect of my body that was out of alignment. If I can do it, so can you, too!

I have shifted into a space where there is no attachment to outcome. I have embraced everything about myself. Operating from a place of authenticity is a beautiful place to be. Fears and self-doubt have been replaced by a deep knowing and neutrality. My heart has become unconditional for self and others. The past is just a reminder that it was just an experience and somehow all these experiences needed to play out exactly the way they did. Sometimes who we think we are is a distortion. Most of us are a rendition of our family lineage, ancestry, and pain-bodies. A big percentage of who we are is just another version of our families' patterns. Remove these patterns and you will see who you truly are and what you are capable of. We are Infinite brilliance and an aspect of Pure Source. Manifesting will come from a place of knowing that we already have everything we want. The Universe works for us. You become so aligned with your Soul, Spirit, and Pure Source that you will automatically follow your heart and know what you came here to do. One of the things I truly learned and embraced through my healing is to stop playing small. I stopped giving my power away. I AM no longer living my life through the expectations of others. The decision to let go and shift healed my family lineage and ancestral lines as well. There is no separation. We are all one and energetically connected. I accepted that the turmoil growing up and the two near-death experiences at an early age were already in preparation for what was to come.

Another Divine intervention saved my life from a head-on collision in my mid-twenties. These near-death experiences brought me into a "no space and time" so I could receive the upgrades and downloads necessary. The process of shifting, empowering, and healing was beautiful and challenging at times. Not everyone is going to like the new and empowered you, and that is okay. It is your journey, not theirs. Not everyone is going to like the new frequency you are operating from. Your authentic, high vibration, and frequency may trigger a lot of old stuff within others.

The act of Loving ourselves is an act of courage. We often mirror back and forth the unhealed parts within ourselves. We also reflect back the healed parts. This will bring in a whole new Soul tribe and friendships that are like minded. Energy never lies.

I realized that the only one who was ever critical of me was ME. Once you make up your mind, the Universe and your Soul will open up to possibilities you never imagined. You will be rewarded. For the past fifteen years I have stepped back into my Soul purpose to serve in awakening Humanity. I have shared my unique Soul Signature, insights, work, gifts, and abilities with clients all over the world, and I will continue to do so until my last breath. I knew from a very young age that my soul's purpose here is to bring a deeper understanding of our true purpose. It is my wish that my experience reaches people at a deeper level, triggering and igniting a recognition of their own divinity, opening their souls to a higher level of consciousness and personal freedom.

My quantum-frequency work is meant to assist you in releasing your attachment to emotional pain. Replace your fears with the energy of your Infinite Knowing. Heighten your senses to match the frequency of who you truly are.

Awaken portions of the brain that are meant to assist you in tuning into higher dimensional frequencies—connecting you to your Infinite Soul and looking at what you agreed to take on and what the soul's higher self's direction is. Removing old programs, previous lifetimes, frequencies, and old belief systems that no longer serve with the focus on understanding your true human nature and living your authentic self as it was meant to be.

My personal advice to anyone who is ready to shift into their self-healing is this: Don't wait! The time is now! There is so much support out there! More and more people are questioning their life's purpose and being pushed from within to explore and understand a higher aspect of themselves. This will lead them to an awareness of the beliefs and programs that have been running them. This in turn also creates a desire to release these limiting beliefs and programs so they can live at a higher level of personal freedom.

Now is the time to delve deeper into your own journey of self-discovery! With the supportive energies propelling us forward and the nudge we are receiving from within, it's now time to take action. Uncover the True You! Align with the frequencies of success, abundance, and prosperity on all levels. People have reported profound changes as a result of the clarity and understanding gained regarding their direction and purpose. It is empowering to see yourself as a beautiful proactive being, allowing yourself to access your soul purpose and transmute all that no longer serves. Suffering will be a thing in the past! We are whole and made of light. We all have access to that same infinite pure source light. That is our birthright.

I AM living proof that when we change our perspectives, we change our lives. Each Soul without exception has a goal, a reason for creating this life experience. My group of amazing guides encourage me to continue to say yes to God/Pure Source and yes to every experience to become more empowered and of service. My work is neither religious nor spiritual. I have no attachment to anything organized and wish to lead from a place of knowing, freedom, neutrality, and connection to all that is. May you discover a heart filled with unconditional love for self and others. May you also continually grow, expand, and awaken to your highest potential. We are here to find and connect to our Divine spark again. I wish you Happiness.

Love,

Win

RESOURCES

Products
- Frankie's: Gluten-free baked products, https://glutenfreefrankies.com/
- Juice Plus+: Whole-food-based nutrition in a capsule, https://nicolescott.canada.juiceplus.com/
- Loren Lahav's *I Am cards:* https://www.i-am-cards.com/daily-life-changing-affirmations
- Olaplex: Products that protect the hair from damage from hot styling tools, and other hair products, https://olaplex.com/

Toxin-free Businesses
- Energy Organic Salon, Newmarket, Ontario, https://www.energyorganicsalon.com
- Green Beaver Company, Hawkesbury, Ontario, https://greenbeaver.com/en
- Green Hair Zone, Newmarket, Ontario, http://www.greenhairzone.ca/
- Henna Hair Salon, Whitby, Ontario, https://www.hennahairsalon.com/
- Herbatint, https://ca.herbatint.com/en

- O&M Australian Born Hair Care, https://www.originalmineral.com/
- Organic Color Systems, UK, https://www.organiccolorsystems.com/

Practitioner and General Information Websites

- Adriana Girdler, Cornerstone Dynamics: Business Productivity Specialists, https://www.cornerstonedynamics.com/adriana-girdler/
- Caroline Marie Dupont, Soul Coach, Meditation and Yoga Teacher, and Holistic Nutritionist: https://www.carolinedupont.com/
- Dr. Mitra Ray: http://www.drmitraray.com/
- Environmental Working Group (EWG) guides: https://www.ewg.org/
- Environmental Working Group (EWG) Skin Deep Cosmetics Database: https://www.ewg.org/skindeep/site/about.php
- Government of Canada's "Cosmetic Ingredient Hotlist" for a list of prohibited or restricted ingredients in cosmetic products: https://www.canada.ca/en/health-canada/services/consumer-product-safety/cosmetics/cosmetic-ingredient-hotlist-prohibited-restricted-ingredients/hotlist.html
- Instructions for using henna for hair, Ancient Sunrise, https://www.mehandi.com/Articles.asp?ID=257
- Jenn Pike, Registered Holistic Nutritionist, specializing in women's health and hormones, https://jennpike.com
- Made Safe, a website to help you avoid toxins in products from personal care to household items, https://www.madesafe.org/
- My Gorgeous Grey Movement: Women Inspiring Women to Own Their Grey Sparkle on Facebook: https://www.facebook.com/groups/250601575656819

- Nicole Scott's "Own Your Sparkle" Facebook page: https://business.facebook.com/ownyoursparklemovement/?business_id=206811609348103 8
- Nicole Scott's "Own Your Sparkle" Instagram page: https://www.instagram.com/own_your_sparkle/
- Nicole Scott's "Own Your Sparkle" website: www.nicolescott.ca
- Samantha Gladish, Holistic Nutritionist, guides women in holistic wellness, https://holisticwellness.ca/
- The DNA Company: DNA testing to learn what the best diet and supplements would be best for you: https://www.thednacompany.com/home
- Wineke (Winnie) Engelage, Owner/Operator at Core Soul: https://core-soul.com/home
- Zac Lioutas, Spirtitual Elder, Master Key Holder, Soul Activator, and Meditation Teacher: https://www.zaklioutas.com/

Books

Chapman, Gary, *The 5 Love Languages: The Secret to Love that Lasts*. Northfield Publishing, Chicago, IL: 2015.

Deacon, Gillian, *There's Lead in Your Lipstick: Toxins in Our Everyday Body Care and How to Avoid Them*. Penguin Group (Canada), Toronto: 2011.

Epstein, Samuel S., *Toxic Beauty: How Cosmetics and Personal-Care Products Endanger Your Health … and What You Can Do about It*. BenBella Books, Dallas, TX: 2009.

Grace, Annie, *This Naked Mind: Control Alcohol, Find Freedom, Discover Happiness & Change Your Life*. Avery, New York: 2018.

Hay, Louise, *You Can Heal Your Life*. Hay House, Carlsbad, CA: *1984*.

Jensen, Karen, and Marita Schauch, *The Adrenal Stress Connection. Mind Publishing, Coquitlam, BC: 2015*.

Malkan, Stacey, *Not Just a Pretty Face: The Ugly Side of the Beauty Industry*. New Society Publishers, Gabriola Island, BC: 2007.

Ray, Mitra and Jennifer Daniels, *Do You Have the Guts to Be Beautiful?* Shining Star Publishing, Seattle, WA: 2008.

Russ, Elle, *The Paleo Thyroid Solution: Stop Feeling Fat, Foggy, and Fatigued at the Hands of Uninformed Doctors. Primal Blueprint Publishing, Oxnard, CA: 2016*.

Williamson, Marianne, *A Return to Love: Reflections on the Principles of A Course in Miracles. HarperCollins, New York: 1996*.

NOTES

Chapter One

[1] Mayo Clinic, with Yvonne Butler Tobah, MD, "Is It OK to Use Hair Dye During Pregnancy?" July 13, 2017, accessed November 3, 2019, https://www.mayoclinic.org/healthy-lifestyle/pregnancy-week-by-week/expert-answers/hair-dye-and-pregnancy/faq-20058484.

[2] National Health Service, UK, "Is It Safe to Use Hair Dye When I'm Pregnant or Breastfeeding?" May 3, 2018, accessed November 3, 2019, https://www.nhs.uk/common-health-questions/pregnancy/is-it-safe-to-use-hair-dye-when-i-am-pregnant-or-breastfeeding/.

[3] Paul Cahalan, "Hair Dye That Can Harm a Woman's Fertility and Endanger Unborn Babies is Banned," February 7, 2016, accessed November 3, 2019, https://www.dailymail.co.uk/news/article-3435432/Hair-dye-harm-woman-s-fertility-endanger-unborn-babies-banned.html.

[4] American Pregnancy Association, "Hair Treatment During Pregnancy: Is It Safe?" October 11, 2019, accessed November 3, 2091, https://americanpregnancy.org/is-it-safe/hair-treatments-during-pregnancy/.

[5] Julia Brucculieri, HuffPost US, "Is Dyeing Your Hair When You're Pregnant Really That Bad? Doctors Weigh In." April 29, 2019, accessed November 3, 2019, https://

www.huffingtonpost.ca/entry/hair-dye-during-pregnanc y_n_5abcf8aee4b04a59a3154eb3.

6 Environmental Working Group, "Body Burden: The pollution in Newborns," July 14, 2005, accessed September 13, 2019, https://www.ewg.org/research/body-burden-pollution-newborns. Copyright © Environmental Working Group, www.ewg.org. Reproduced with permission.

7 Jasmine A. McDonald et al., "Alcohol Intake and Breast Cancer Risk: Weighing the Overall Evidence," *Current Breast Cancer Reports* 5, no. 3 (2013). doi:10.1007/ s12609-013-0114-z.

8 ScienceDaily, "Higher Estrogen Levels Linked to Increased Alcohol Sensitivity in Brain's 'Reward Center,'" November 7, 2017, accessed September 15, 2019, https://www.sciencedaily. com/releases/2017/11/171107092906.htm.

9 American Cancer Society, "Alcohol Use and Cancer," April 5, 2017, accessed September 15, 2019, https://www.cancer.org/cancer/ cancer-causes/diet-physical-activity/alcohol-use-and-cancer.html.

10 American Cancer Society, "Alcohol Use and Cancer."

11 McDonald, "Alcohol Intake and Breast Cancer Risk."

12 Alexandra Gerea "Your Nail Polish Might Be Toxic. Here's How You Can Tell," April 29, 2019, accessed September 15, 2019, https://www.zmescience.com/science/domestic-science/ nail-polish-toxic/.

13 Heather White, "Your Nail Polish Could be Disrupting Your Hormone System," October 21, 2015, accessed September 15, 2019, https://www.ewg.org/enviroblog/2015/10/ your-nail-polish-could-be-disrupting-your-hormone-system.

14 American Academy of Dermatology, "Gel Manicures: The Good, the Bad and the UV," February 2, 2016, accessed September 15, 2019, https://www.aad.org/media/news-releases/ gel-manicures-dermatologists-share-tips-to-keep-nails-healthy.

15 Made Safe, "How to Avoid Toxic Chemicals in Plastics," December 13, 2016, accessed September 15, 2019, https://www.madesafe.org/avoid-toxic-chemicals-plastics/.

16 John Hamilton, "Study: Most Plastics Leach Hormone-Like Chemicals," March 2, 2011, accessed September 15, 2019, https://www.npr.org/2011/03/02/134196209/study-most-plastics-leach-hormone-like-chemicals.

Chapter Two

1 Marshall Brain, "How Hair Coloring Works," 2019, accessed September 17, 2019, https://science.howstuffworks.com/innovation/everyday-innovations/hair-coloring.htm.

2 Private Label Extensions, "What You Didn't Know about Hair Color throughout American History," 2019, accessed September 17, 2019, https://www.privatelabelextensions.com/hair-color-american-history/.

3 YouTube, "100 Years of Hair Color," n.d., accessed September 18, 2019, https://www.youtube.com/watch?v=6jizLusbRkY.

4 Devon Hopp, "From 1500 BC to 2015 AD: The Extraordinary History of Hair Color," May 5, 2019, accessed September 18, 2019, https://www.byrdie.com/hair-color-history/slide8.

5 Taylor Stephan and Diana Nguyen, "A Brief History of Hair Coloring and Dye Trends—From Coal Tar to Unicorn Tresses," August 3, 2015, accessed September 18, 2019, https://www.eonline.com/ca/news/682836/a-brief-history-of-hair-coloring-and-dye-trends-from-coal-tar-to-unicorn-tresses.

6 Vivian Diller, "Graying: Is the Double Standard Diminishing? May 31, 2011, accessed September 18, 2019, https://www.psychologytoday.com/ca/blog/face-it/201105/graying-is-the-double-standard-diminishing.

7 Wikipedia, "List of Countries by Life Expectancy," 2015, accessed September 18, 2019, https://en.wikipedia.org/wiki/List_of_countries_by_life_expectancy.

8 Mark DeWolf, U.S. Department of Labor Blog, "12 Stats about Working Women," March 1, 2017, accessed September 18, 2019, https://blog.dol.gov/2017/03/01/12-stats-about-working-women.

9 Statistics Canada, "Fewer Children, Older Moms," May 17, 2018, accessed September 20, 2019, https://www150.statcan.gc.ca/n1/pub/11-630-x/11-630-x2014002-eng.htm.

10 Claudine Provenher, et al., Statistics Canada, "Fertility: Overview, 2012 to 2016," June 5, 2018, accessed September 18, 2019, https://www150.statcan.gc.ca/n1/pub/91-209-x/2018001/article/54956-eng.htm.

11 Grand View Research, "Hair Care Market Size Worth $211.1 Billion by 2025," March 2018, accessed September 18, 2019, https://www.grandviewresearch.com/press-release/global-hair-care-market.

12 Goldstein Research, "Hair Color Market and Forecast (2016–2024)," n.d., accessed September 20, 2019, https://www.goldsteinresearch.com/report/global-hair-color-market-outlook-2024-global-opportunity-and-demand-analysis-market-forecast-2016-2024.

13 Jennifer Chait, "Who Buys Organic Food: Different Types of Consumers," January 14, 2019, accessed September 18, 2019, https://www.thebalancesmb.com/who-buys-organic-food-different-types-of-consumers-2538042.

14 Government of Canada, "Canadian Cancer Statistics: Highlights of What You Will Find in the Canadian Cancer Statistics 2017 Annual Report," October 23, 2017, accessed September 18, 2019, https://www.canada.ca/en/

public-health/services/chronic-diseases/cancer/canadian-cancer-statistics.html.

15 Kelly Atterton, "What Does the Future of Beauty Look Like?" July 6, 2015, accessed September 18, 2019, https://www.allure.com/story/beauty-technology-leslie-blodgett.

16 Joanna Mazewski, "L'Oreal and Vogue Declare Grey Hair the Hottest Shade of the Year," April 4, 2019, accessed September 18, 2019, https://www.moms.com/grey-hair-the-shade-of-the-year-how-to-achieve-the-look/?utm_content=buffer1f82e&utm_medium=Social-Distribution&utm_source=MM-FB-P&utm_campaign=MM-FB-P&fbclid=IwAR1HUQpmbnWprnq2_O38nYZX1ULKwiScd9jMvtVgOFcSb7bhPRs4ni6v9qs.

17 Joanne Mazewski, "L'Oreal and Vogue."

18 Devon Abelman, "Gray Hair Is Set to Be 2018's Most Popular Hair-Color Trend," January 5, 2018, accessed September 18, 2019, https://www.allure.com/story/tracing-the-gray-hair-trend.

19 Anne Kreamer, "The War Over Going Gray," August 31, 2007, accessed September 20, 2019, https://content.time.com/time/nation/article/0,8599,1658058-2,00.html.

20 Anne Kreamer, "The War Over Going Gray."

Chapter Three

1 EWG's Skin Deep Cosmetics Database, n.d., accessed September 23, 2019, https://www.ewg.org/skindeep/site/about.php.

2 National Institute of Environmental Health Sciences, "Endocrine Disruptors," n.d., accessed September 25,

2019, https://www.niehs.nih.gov/health/materials/endocrine_disruptors_508.pdf.

3 Chris Brooke, "Coroner Attacks Cosmetics Firms after Mother Died of Massive Allergic Reaction to her L'Oréal Hair Dye," *Daily Mail*, UK, February 19, 2015, accessed September 23, 2019.

4 Wendy Gillis, "Hair Dye Ingredient Linked to Coma, Death," *The Star*, November 22, 1019, accessed September 23, 2019, https://www.thestar.com/life/health_wellness/news_research/2011/11/22/hair_dye_ingredient_linked_to_coma_death.html.

5 The Belgravia Centre Blog, "Petition Launched to Ban PPD Hair Dye Chemical in UK," n.d., accessed September 23, 2019, https://www.belgraviacentre.com/blog/petition-launched-to-ban-ppd-hair-dye-chemical-in-uk/.

6 Timo Leino et al., "Occurrence of Asthma and Chronic Bronchitis Among Female Hairdressers: A Questionnaire Study," *Journal of Occupational and Environmental Medicine* 39, no. 6 (June 1997): 534-539.

7 Timo Leino et al., "Working Conditions and Health in Hairdressing Salons," *Journal of Applied Occupational and Environmental Hygiene* 14, no. 1 (1999): 26-33.

8 Gianna Moscato and Eugenia Galdi, "Asthma and Hairdressers," *Current Opinion in Allergy and Clinical Immunology* 6, no. 2 (2006): 91-95.

9 Andrew D. Blainey et al., "Occupational Asthma in a Hairdressing Salon," *Thorax* 41, no. 1 (January 1986): 42-50.

10 Nathaniel Shafer and Robert W. Shafer, "Potential of Carcinogenic Effects of Hair Dyes," *New York State Journal of Medicine* 76, no. 3 (1976): 394-396.

11 Chisato Nagata et al., "Hair Dye Use and Occupational Exposure to Organic Solvents as Risk Factors for

Myelodysplastic Syndrome," *Leukemia Research* 23, no. 1 (January 1999): 57-62.

[12] Paolo Boffetta et al., "Employment as Hairdresser and Risk of Ovarian Cancer and Non-Hodgkin's Lymphomas among Women, *Journal of Occupational Medicine and Toxicology* 36, no. 1 (1994): 61-55.

[13] Manuela Gago-Dominguez et al., "Use of Permanent Hair Dyes and Bladder-Cancer Risk," *International Journal of Cancer* 15, no. 4 (2001): 575-579.

[14] Anastasia Tzonou et al., "Hair Dyes, Analgesics, Tranquilizers and Perineal Talk Application as Risk Factors for Ovarian Cancer," *International Journal of Cancer* 30, no. 55 (September 1993): 408-410.

[15] Sanna Heikkinen et al., "Does Hair Dye Use Increase the Risk of Breast Cancer? A Population-Based Case-Control Study of Finnish Women," *PLoS ONE* 10, no. 8 (August 2015): e0135190.

[16] Adana A.M. Llanos et al., "Use of Dark Hair Dye and Relaxers Associated with Increased Breast Cancer Risk," June 14, 2017, accessed September 24, 2019, https://cinj.org/use-dark-hair-dye-and-relaxers-associated-increased-breast-cancer-risk.

[17] Peter Saitta et al., "Is There a True Concern Regarding the Use of Hair Dye and Malignancy Development: A Review of the Epidemiological Evidence Relating Personal Hair Dye Use to the Risk of Malignancy," *Journal of Clinical Aesthetic Dermatology* 6, no. 1 (January 2013): 39-46.

[18] Gabriella M. Johansson et al., "Exposure of Hairdressers to Ortho- and Meta-Toluidine in Hair Dyes," 72 (2015):57-63.

[19] American Cancer Society, "Hair Dyes," May 27, 2014, accessed September 24, 2019, https://www.cancer.org/cancer/cancer-causes/hair-dyes.html.

[20] American Cancer Society, "Hair Dyes."

[21] The Medical Station, "The Medical Station Explores the Dangers of Hair Dyes, n.d., accessed September 24, 2019, https://www.themedicalstation. com/site/blog-doctor-north-york/2016/03/07/ medical-clinic-explores-dangers-of-hair-dyes.

[22] National Capital Poison Center, "Concern about Hair Dye: Prevent Injuries and Allergic Reactions," c.2016, accessed September 24, 2019, https://www.poison.org/ articles/2016-sep/hair-dye.

[23] Graham Smith, "Schoolgirl Blinded by Hair Dye wins £20,000 Payout," *Daily Mail*, UK, December 1, 2009, accessed September 24, 2019, https://www.dailymail.co.uk/ news/article-1232398/Schoolgirl-blinded-hair-dye-wins-20-000-payout.html.

[24] Poison Control, "Concern about Hair Dye.

[25] Hannah McGrath, "Wembley Barrister 'Lucky to Be Alive' after Suffering Allergic Reaction to Hair Dye," *Brent & Kilburn Times*, September 8, 2015, accessed September 24, 2019, https://www.kilburntimes.co.uk/news/wembley-barrister-lucky-to-be-alive-after-suffering-allergic-reaction-to-hair-dye-1-4216582.

[26] Makeda A. Drew, "Dying Due to Dye," December 4, 2015, accessed September 24, 2019, https://sites.psu.edu/ siowfa15/2015/12/04/dying-due-to-dye/.

[27] Michelle Kmiec, "Europe Bans Food Dyes Due to ADHD & Cancer Links, April 19, 2013, accessed September 24, 2019, http://csglobe.com/ europe-bans-food-dyes-due-to-adhd-cancer-links/.

[28] New Hampshire Public Radio, "Why M&M's Are Made with Natural Coloring in the EU and not the U.S.," n.d., accessed September 25, 2019, https://www.nhpr.org/

post/why-mms-are-made-natural-coloring-eu-and-not-us#stream/0.

29 Janice Melanson, "The Story of Cosmetics – What's Canada's Story?" 2016, accessed September 25, 2019, http://www.preventcancernow.ca/the-story-of-cosmetics-%E2%80%93-what%E2%80%99s-canada%E2%80%99s-story/.

30 Government of Canada, "Cosmetic Ingredient Hotlist: List of Ingredients that Are Prohibited for Use in Cosmetic Products," June 14, 2018, accessed September 24, 2019, https://www.canada.ca/en/health-canada/services/consumer-product-safety/cosmetics/cosmetic-ingredient-hotlist-prohibited-restricted-ingredients/hotlist.html.

31 Janice Melanson, "The Story of Cosmetics."

32 SciNews, "Scientists Categorize Earth as a 'Toxic Planet,'" February 7, 2017, accessed September 24, 2019, https://phys.org/news/2017-02-scientists-categorize-earth-toxic-planet.html.

33 Sam Escobar, "How Young Is Too Young to Dye Your Kid's Hair?" *Good Housekeeping*, October 15, 2018, accessed September 24, 2019, https://www.goodhousekeeping.com/beauty/hair/a38165/how-young-is-too-young-to-color-hair/.

Chapter Four

1 Reprinted with some editing with permission from Energy Organic Salon.

2 Reprinted with some editing with permission from Green Hair Zone.

3 Reprinted with some editing with permission from Henna Hair Salon.

4 Reprinted with some editing with permission from Organic Colour Systems.

5 Reprinted with some editing with permission from O&M.

6 Reprinted with some editing with permission from Bioforce Canada Inc., makers of Herbatint.

7 Reprinted with some editing with permission from Alain Ménard, Co-founder, The Green Beaver Company.

8 Reprinted with some editing with permission from Mitra Ray.

9 Pooja Karkala, "10 Best Organic Hair Colors to Try in 1=2019," May 20, 2019, accessed September 30, 2019, https://www.stylecraze.com/articles/best-organic-hair-color-brands/.

Chapter Five

1 Michael Melnychuk et al., "Coupling of Respiration and Attention via the Locus Coeruleus: Effects of Meditation and Pranayama," *Psychophysiology* 55, no. 3 (2018). doi:10.1111/psyp.13091.

2 Steven M. Toepfer, Kelly Cichy, and Patti Peters, "Letters of Gratitude: Further Evidence of Author Benefits," *Journal of Happiness Studies* 13, no. 1 (2012):187-201.

3 Marianne Williamson, *A Return to Love: Reflections on the Principles of A Course in Miracles* (New York: HarperCollins, 1996), 190-191. Reprinted, along with the quotation at beginning of this chapter, with permission from The Williamson Institute.

Chapter Six

1 Michael Colgan, *Optimum Sports Nutrition: Your Competitive Edge* (Ronkonkoma, NY: Advanced Research Press, 1993).

2 Matthew Hoffman, "Picture of the Hair," *Web*MD, n.d., accessed October 4, 2019, https://www.webmd.com/skin-problems-and-treatments/picture-of-the-hair#1.

3 Kaustubh Adhikari, et al., "A Genome-wide Association Scan in Admixed Latin Americans Identifies Loci Influencing Facial and Scalp Hair Features," *Nature Communications* 7:10815 (2016). doi:10.1038/ncomms10815.

4 Adhikari, "A Genome-wide Association."

5 Imperial College London, "Eating Up to Ten Portions of Fruit and Vegetables a Day May Prevent 7.8 Million Premature Deaths Worldwide," *ScienceDaily*, February 23, 2017, accessed October 7, 2019, https://www.sciencedaily.com/releases/2017/02/170223102404.htm.

6 Katya Slepian, "Canadians Eating Fewer Fruits, Veggies Compared to 11 Years Ago: Study," *The Columbia Valley Pioneer*, February 25, 2019, accessed October 7, 2019, https://www.columbiavalleypioneer.com/trending-now/canadians-eating-fewer-fruits-veggies-compared-to-11-years-ago-study/.

7 Centers for Disease Control and Prevention, "Only 1 in 10 Adults Get Enough Fruits or Vegetables," November 16, 2017, accessed October 7, 2019, https://www.cdc.gov/media/releases/2017/p1116-fruit-vegetable-consumption.html.

8 Linus Pauling Institute, Micronutrient Information Center, "Essential Fatty Acids," n.d., accessed October 8, 2019, https://lpi.oregonstate.edu/mic/other-nutrients/essential-fatty-acids.

9 Sherry Torkos and Karolyn A. Gazella, "Essential Fatty Acids and Antioxidants Benefit Women with Female Pattern Hair Loss: Hair Growth and Density Improve with Supplementation," *Natural Medicine Journal* 7,

no. 4 (2015), accessed October 8, 2019, https://www.naturalmedicinejournal.com/journal/2015-04/essential-fatty-acids-and-antioxidants-benefit-women-female-pattern-hair-loss.

10 Kellie Langlois and Walisundera M.N. Ratnayake, Statistics Canada, "Omega-3 Index of Canadian Adults," November 27, 2015, accessed October 8, 2019, https://www150.statcan.gc.ca/n1/pub/82-003-x/2015011/article/14242-eng.htm.

11 Yanni Papanikolaou et al., "U.S. Adults Are Not Meeting Recommended Levels for Fish and Omega-3 Fatty Acid Intake: Results of an Analysis Using Observational Data from NHANES 2003–2008," *Nutrition Journal* 13, no. 1 (2014): 31.

12 Robert L. Mort, Ian J. Jackson, and E. Elizabeth Patton, "The Melanocyte Lineage in Development and Disease," *Development* 142 (2015): 620-632.

13 Ayman A. Zayed et al., "Smokers' Hair: Does Smoking Cause Premature Hair Graying?" *Indian Dermatology Online Journal* 4, no. 2 (2013): 90-92. Accessed October 8, 2019, https://www.ncbi.nlm.nih.gov/pmc/articles/PMC3673399/.

14 Hyoseung Shin et al., "Association of Premature Hair Graying with Family History, Smoking, and Obesity: A Cross-Sectional Study," *Journal American Academy of Dermatology* 72, no. 2 (2015): 321-327.

15 Wei Chin Chou et al., "Direct Migration of Follicular Melanocyte Stem Cells to the Epidermis after Wounding or UVB Irradiation is Dependent on Mc1r Signaling," *Nature Medicine* 19 (2013): 924-929.

16 Coco Ballantyne, "Fact of Fiction? Stress Causes Gray Hair," *Scientific American*, October 24, 2007, accessed October 8, 2019, https://www.scientificamerican.com/article/fact-or-fiction-stress-causes-gray-hair/.

[17] J. Jaime Miranda et al., "Hair Follicle Characteristics as Early Marker of Type 2 Diabetes," *Medical Hypotheses* 95 (2016): 39-44.

[18] Ségolène Panhard, Isabelle Lozano, and Geneviève Loussouarn, "Greying of the Human Hair: A Worldwide Survey, Revisiting the '50' Rule of Thumb," *British Journal of Dermatology* 167, no. 3 (2012): 865-873.

[19] Jennifer Berry, "Benefits and Uses of B-Complex Vitamins," April 1, 2019, accessed October 9, 2019, https://www.medicalnewstoday.com/articles/324856.php.

[20] National Institutes of Health, "Omega-3 Fatty Acids," November 21, 2018, accessed October 9, 2019, https://ods.od.nih.gov/factsheets/Omega3FattyAcids-Consumer/.

[21] Ségolène Panhard, Isabelle Lozano, and Geneviève Loussouarn, "Greying of the Human Hair: A Worldwide Survey, Revisiting the '50' Rule of Thumb," British Journal of Dermatology 167, no. 3 (2012): 865-873

Chapter Eight

[1] Merriam-Webster, "Definition of *brave*," n.d., accessed October 14, 2019, https://www.merriam-webster.com/dictionary/brave.

[2] Karen Jensen and Marita Schauch, The Adrenal Stress Connection (Coquitlam, BC: Mind Publishing, 2015). Reprinted with permission from Karen Jensen and Marita Schauch.

ABOUT THE AUTHOR

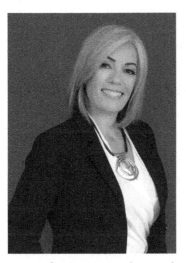

Nicole Scott is a Holistic Nutritionist, Healthy Lifestyle Expert, Author, International Wellness speaker, Network Marketing Professional and a mom of 2 teenage girls who lives in the Greater Toronto area in Canada.

Nicole graduated from the University of Calgary with a BA in Psychology and Business minor. She worked for 10 years in the food manufacturing industry before changing careers after learning her daughter had food allergies, which inspired her to change careers. After graduating in 2005 from the Canadian School of Natural Nutrition, she worked in a wellness clinic, consulting and teaching nutrition workshops in her community. That changed when her mother introduced her to Juice Plus, a product line focused on plant based solutions. Having a passion for business and nutrition, she bought a wellness franchise which was a perfect fit for a home-based business with 2 young children. Nicole achieved the top position of National Marketing Director "100 club member" with the Juice Plus Company while staying home raising her children. Nicole is truly following her dreams and living life to the PLUS. She is dedicated to improving the HEALTH of families and she does this by: speaking to audiences around the world, educating on social media, offering a healthy lifestyle program and leading a group of passionate health warriors around the world.

The Gorgeous Grey Movement came to be after a health scare she experienced in 2018. Nicole found two lumps in her breast, and this led her on a path to discovery. That panic of "what if" set in. The lumps were only cysts, but this was a big wake-up call for her to dig deep and examine her lifestyle choices. On her healing journey she discovered how dangerous the toxins were that she was using monthly to dye her dark hair. She knew it was time to detox her body and attain better health. This led her to create the Gorgeous Grey Movement and inspire others to join her in "Owning Your Sparkle." Over the last decade, Nicole has mentored thousands of women to take their health and lives to the next level.

Nicole's wish for this movement is to empower more women to come out of the closet with their *Grey Sparkle* and *own* it—for the health of it!

CONNECT WITH ME

Website www.nicolescott.ca

FB group https://www.facebook.com/
groups/250601575656819/
(Gorgeous Grey Movement)

Instagram https://www.instagram.com/own_your_sparkle/

LinkedIn https://www.linkedin.com/in/ownyoursparkle/

Made in the USA
Monee, IL
10 June 2020